Pulmonary and Respiratory Diseases and Disorders

AF764765

nova
Medicine & Health
New York

Pulmonary and Respiratory Diseases and Disorders

Interstitial Lung Disease: From Diagnosis to Treatment
Roberto G. Carbone, MD, FCCP,
Francesco Puppo, MD,
Keith Wille, MD, MSPH,
Pallav Shah, MD (Editors)
2022. ISBN: 978-1-68507-926-0 (Hardcover)
2022. ISBN: 979-8-88697-068-5 (eBook)

A Clinical Manual of Sarcoidosis
Shambhu Aryal, MD, Vikas Pathak, MD (Editors)
2022. ISBN: 978-1-68507-681-8 (Hardcover)
2022. ISBN: 978-1-68507-782-2 (eBook)

Pulmonary Vascular Disorders
Roberto G. Carbone, MD, FCCP,
Francesco Puppo, MD,
Victor F. Tapson, MD, FCCP, FRCP (Editors)
2021. ISBN: 978-1-53619-458-6 (Hardcover)
2021. ISBN: 978-1-53619-553-8 (eBook)

Non-Invasive Mechanical Ventilation Complications: Essentials for Treatment and Prevention
Antonio M. Esquinas, M.D, Ph.D (Editor)
2021. ISBN: 978-1-53619-515-6 (Hardcover)
2021. ISBN: 978-1-53619-903-1 (eBook)

More information about this series can be found at
https://novapublishers.com/product-category/series/pulmonary-and-respiratory-diseases-and-disorders/

James K. Edwards
Editor

Understanding and Treating Acute Pulmonary Embolism

Medicine & Health
New York

Library of Congress Cataloging-in-Publication Data

ISBN: 979-8-88697-149-1

Published by Nova Science Publishers, Inc. † New York

Contents

Preface

This book contains five chapters, each focusing on an aspect of understanding and treating acute Pulmonary embolism. Chapter One is an overview of the state of the science regarding the treatment of acute pulmonary embolism, and provides modern insights into recent developments. The second chapter reviews a novel technology for the detection and diagnosis of pulmonary embolism which may provide benefits over currently used technologies. The third chapter is a wide-ranging review of the state of clinical practice in diagnosing pulmonary embolism prior to the COVID-19 pandemic in Southern Spain. Chapter Four provides a systematic review of the use of ultrasound-assisted catheter-directed thrombolysis in treating acute pulmonary embolism. The final chapter discusses the issue of subsegmental pulmonary embolism, and whether it should be treated directly.

Chapter 1 - Acute pulmonary embolism (PE) poses grave morbidity and mortality risks as sudden obstruction by an embolus in the pulmonary vasculature can lead to rapid cardiovascular collapse. Appropriate measures must be taken to minimize complications. This study follows updated guidelines from the American Heart Association and European Society of Cardiology, comparing each recommendation in terms of the latest management data, evidence level, and strength. Sources were further analyzed and evaluated to obtain relevant information. In the study, researchers found that similar recommendations proposed by both guidelines sometimes had different levels of evidence or strength, posing interesting questions for critical review. Furthermore, in some cases, recommendations provided by one guideline were not mentioned by the other, and vice versa. These differences show the importance of reviewing the literature in order to gain insight into the underlying reason for every recommendation. Therefore, this chapter enables understanding of the proposed guidelines based on the current research available in the field of acute PE management.

Chapter 2 - Computed tomography pulmonary angiography (CTPA) is the imaging technique of choice for the diagnosis of pulmonary embolism (PE).

In clinical practice, multidetector single-energy CT (SECT) is the most commonly used worldwide. Dual-energy computed tomography (DECT) is a novel technology increasingly used in clinical practice. DECT offers different imaging postprocessing techniques based on the advantages of dual energy acquisition (e.g., linear blending, iodine maps, and virtual monoenergetic reconstructions) which maximize differences in contrast attenuation of tissues. This can aid in the diagnosis of PE. In this chapter, the authors report an up-to-date review of current evidence on the efficacy and possible advantages of DECT in the diagnosis of PE. The authors conducted a systematic review following the PRISMA guidelines. The authors performed structures searches in the main medical databases (PubMed, Web of Science, Scopus, Cochrane). The authors included observational studies, trials and systematic reviews analyzing the effectiveness of DECT in PE detection, contrast material used, and ionizing radiation rates. The authors' results indicate that DECT and SECT yield similar sensitivity and specificity values regarding PE detection. DECT allows the administration of a lower volume of iodine contrast agents and implies lower ionizing radiation. However, further studies are required to determine its cost-effectiveness compared to DECT.

Chapter 3 - The aim of this study was to evaluate the use of clinical probability scores and several factors related to the diagnosis of pulmonary embolism (PE) in patients that underwent computed tomography chest angiography (CTCA) for suspected PE at the emergency department (ED) in the authors' institution. Retrospective observational study addressing the CTCAs ordered for suspected PE in the authors' ED during 2018. Epidemiological, clinical and analytical factors, as well as the use of clinical probability scores (CPS), were analyzed. Two-level Wells score (WS), revised Geneva score (GS) and their simplified versions (sWS and sGS, respectively) were retrospectively calculated, and guideline adherence was analyzed accordingly.

In total, 534 patients (52.8% women, median age: 73 years) were included. The frequency of PE was 23.0%. The WS had been explicitly applied in 15.2% of all cases. Significant differences were found between retrospective CPSs (PE likely: WS (12.9%); sWS (26.4%); GS (45.5%); sGS (43.4%); $p < 0.001$). D-dimer tests were ordered in 88.2% of all cases (97.6% and 93.4% were positive, according to the standard and age-adjusted upper limits, respectively). Lack of adherence to guidelines varied between CPSs (WS: 15.6%; sWS: 24.0%; GS: 40.3%; sGS: 39.0%).

In conclusion, a poor explicit use of the WS was observed in the authors' study. The authors' results suggest that the yield of clinical gestalt assessment might be similar to that of CPSs. However, specific studies are further required to verify the authors' findings.

Chapter 4 - Traditionally, acute pulmonary embolism (PE) has been treated with anticoagulation and/or systemic thrombolysis. However, in recent years improvements in interventional therapeutic techniques have facilitated the management of numerous pathologies where conventional therapies are contraindicated or not free of considerable complications. Mechanical or pharmaco-mechanical thrombolysis directed by percutaneous catheter is one of the options available for the treatment of PE and its application is increasing in the emergency department. Ultrasound-assisted catheter-directed thrombolysis (USACDT) is one of the most recently implemented techniques. The aim of this study is to evaluate the efficacy and safety of USACDT for the treatment of PE according to the evidence available to date.

The authors conducted a systematic review by searching the main medical databases. The authors prioritized the inclusion of experimental and observational studies. The authors also reviewed clinical practice guidelines. The authors discuss the different aspects related on the topic according to the available literature.

Current evidence reveals that USACDT is a feasible treatment for PE that reduced mean pulmonary artery pressure and other functional variables, with low risk of major bleeding. Further research is required to determine the most appropriate indications of this treatment.

Chapter 5 - Pulmonary embolism (PE) represents the third leading cause of cardiovascular-related death in the emergency department. Computed tomography pulmonary angiography is the current imaging technique used to diagnose this condition, allowing to detect its location and extension, which may be variable. In fact, these features are essential to determine its severity, along with clinical presentation. It is completely accepted and validated that patients with central forms of PE (i.e., involving the central, main or lobar pulmonary arteries), should receive urgent treatment, either medical or by invasive procedures, depending on PE severity. In the case of more peripheral PEs (i.e., involving subsegmental pulmonary branches), the decision on whether to treat or not is a matter of great controversy in the scientific literature. The aim of this book chapter is to review the studies published on this subject in recent years to determine whether there is current evidence in favor of administering anticoagulation treatment or not in subsegmental forms of PE. To do so, the authors performed a systematic review searching the main medical databases (PubMed, Web of Science, Scopus, Cochrane) and they collected information on clinical trials, systematic reviews or meta-analyses on the topic.

Chapter 1

Updates on the Treatment of Acute Pulmonary Embolism

Andrea Laurentius*, Moira Setiawan, Kelvin Kohar, Aditya Parawangsa and Eric Ferdinand
Faculty of Medicine, Universitas Indonesia,
Central Jakarta, Indonesia

Abstract

Acute pulmonary embolism (PE) poses grave morbidity and mortality risks as sudden obstruction by an embolus in the pulmonary vasculature can lead to rapid cardiovascular collapse. Appropriate measures must be taken to minimize complications. This study follows updated guidelines from the American Heart Association and European Society of Cardiology, comparing each recommendation in terms of the latest management data, evidence level, and strength. Sources were further analyzed and evaluated to obtain relevant information. In the study, researchers found that similar recommendations proposed by both guidelines sometimes had different levels of evidence or strength, posing interesting questions for critical review. Furthermore, in some cases, recommendations provided by one guideline were not mentioned by the other, and vice versa. These differences show the importance of reviewing the literature in order to gain insight into the underlying reason for every recommendation. Therefore, this chapter enables understanding of the proposed guidelines based on the current research available in the field of acute PE management.

---

* Corresponding Author's Email: andrea.laurentius@ui.ac.id.

In: Understanding and Treating Acute Pulmonary Embolism
Editor: James K. Edwards
ISBN: 979-8-88697-149-1

Keywords: acute pulmonary embolism, guideline, management, update

Introduction

Acute pulmonary embolism (PE) is a national health burden, with more than 600,000 cases diagnosed per year, including 100,000 recorded deaths due to the disease in the United States in 2017. This number has been projected to increase from around 142,000 cases per year increase in 21 years. (Turetz et al. 2018) The developing era of radiological medicine has led to the frequent use of computed tomography (CT) scans for diagnosis of acute PE. Now, CT scan is a gold standard for diagnosis of pulmonary embolism following the detection of suspected pulmonary embolism via electrocardiography. (Laurentius and Ariani 2020) The need to improve the effectiveness of PE diagnosis stems from the high level of clinical variability of this condition, ranging from being asymptomatic to causing massive hemodynamic collapse or sudden death. Therefore, it is related to difficulties in respect to diagnosis in the early era of medicine. Considering the severity of the disease, preventing sudden obstruction of an embolus in the pulmonary vasculature, which is an ultimate complication of migrating thrombus dominantly arising from the deep vein of the legs, is widely accepted. (Belicová et al. 2018)

Despite prompt diagnosis and prevention, pulmonary embolism still poses certain grave prognosis. This occurs mainly in patients with multiple comorbidities. Considering its statistics, short-term mortality rates ranged between 17% to 48% within a month and 19% to 30% within a year. (Riedel 2001) Nonetheless, appropriate measures ought to be taken to minimize the risk of morbidity and mortality. Mortality risk increased up to 10-fold in untreated patients than that of patients treated with anticoagulants. The previous guideline encouraged the usage of anticoagulants, such as heparin, for initial treatment of highly suspected pulmonary embolism. Several prominent side effects are noted during the treatment process, such as hemorrhage or thrombocytopenia; therefore, consistent monitoring of hemostatic parameters is widely encouraged. Then, updated research has shown the effectiveness of intravenous thrombolysis as a next-generation treatment for pulmonary embolism. The emergence of mechanical thrombectomy gains superiority against injection of fibrinolytics in terms of systemic bleeding. (Bunc et al. 2020) Research in this field provides insights into better-targeted treatment and minimization of chronic complications and side effects. Recent data and evidence are needed to update the latest recommendations when managing the disease.

Analytical Framework

Literature Review

Acute PE manifests in the rapid deterioration of hemodynamic circulation and gas exchange. Thrombi that block blood flow may be positioned in various branches of the vasculature, according to size. Bigger thrombi predominantly obstruct more proximal and larger vessels, such as the main pulmonary artery. Subsequently, blood flow being pumped directly from the right ventricle eventually does not completely reach the alveolar capillary. Immense blood pressure builds up in the proximal vasculature. This results in acute pulmonary hypertension, causing pressure backflow towards the right ventricle. (Brass et al. 2019) Physiologically, pulmonary vasculature exhibits mechanical vasodilation in response to high blood flow and pressure to accommodate whole lung perfusion. Vasodilation, however, does not fully happen in large pulmonary arteries due to its higher amount of collagen and elastin fibers deposited in their walls. They are specialized in handling the shear stress of ejected blood from the heart. Therefore, obstruction of blood flow in larger arteries may put intense blood pressure back to the right ventricle during systole. The pressure poses stress to the right ventricle's wall and subsequently causes dilation of the chamber. Excessive pressure simultaneously superimposes in outward bulging of interventricular septum toward left ventricle chamber, for right ventricle pressure may counterbalance that of the left ventricle during embolism (Giordano et al. 2017). Decreased left chamber volume during diastole results in lower systemic stroke volume. Thus, increased heart rate compensates to maintain constant cardiac output (Mackman 2012).

Direct obstruction of blood flow in pulmonary vasculature causes ventilation-perfusion mismatch. Minimal blood flow in the alveolar capillaries may impair effective gas exchange. Gas exchange optimally occurs during adequate blood perfusion through the thin alveolar wall, as well as adequate ventilation of air throughout the alveoli; this enables oxygen and carbon dioxide to diffuse back and forth in both alveoli and capillaries based on different partial gas pressures. Obstruction of pulmonary vasculature due to thrombus causes insufficient perfusion of alveoli, thus producing ineffective gas exchange in the lung. It then results in hypoxemia and hypercapnia. Severe hypoxemia ($PaO_2 < 60$ mmHg or $SaO_2 < 88\%$) is one of the risk factors of cardiac arrest (Mata, McDermott, and Diaz 2020; Diamond 2016).

Table 1. Contraindications of fibrinolytic treatment in acute pulmonary embolism

Absolute contraindications	**Relative contraindications**
Active bleeding (excluding menstruation)	Severely uncontrolled hypertension (SBP > 180 mmHg OR DBP > 110 mmHg)
Ischemic stroke < 3 mo.	History of ischemic stroke > 3 mo.
Prior intracranial hemorrhage	Major surgery < 3 wks.
Known cerebral AV malformation	Current use of anticoagulants with INR > 1.7 or PT > 15 secs
Known malignant intracranial neoplasms	Pregnancy
Closed head or facial trauma < 3 mo.	Active peptic ulcer
	Recent internal bleeding 2 – 4 wks.
	Recent invasive procedure
	Pericarditis
	Age > 75 y.o.
	Diabetic retinopathy

In acute PE, the thrombus is composed of aggregated red blood cells and platelets wrapped in a meshwork. The rough surface induces cascades of platelet activation and coagulation factors, contributing to greater aggregation of blood cells into the thrombus. Virchow triads describe the formation of red thrombus in veins, involving blood stasis, hypercoagulability state, and endothelial injury (Ucar 2019). Understanding thrombus formation provides insights into its treatment. Disintegrating fibrin meshwork, preventing platelet aggregation, and inhibiting coagulation factors are three conventional principles of treating acute PE. Because of its hemorrhagic side effect, an invasive procedure is conducted to extract the clogging thrombus or to prevent migration of the thrombus into the lung (Sharifi et al. 2013).

Systemic Fibrinolysis

Systemic fibrinolysis involves the administration of agents that actively dissolve thrombi through the degradation of the fibrin meshwork. These agents convert serum plasminogen into plasmin, which hydrolyzes fibrin polymer into subunits of D-dimer or other fibrin degradation products.

Improvement of hemodynamic circulation and gas exchange are noted following fibrinolysis. Nevertheless, fibrinolysis poses risks of major hemorrhage. The thrombolytic benefit of fibrinolytic agents should therefore outweigh the side effects (bleeding) when used for intermediate- or low-risk patients (Saxena, Smail, and McGiffin 2016). The therapy is effective when applied within the first 48 hours of onset of symptoms; however, efficacy decreases significantly in the period 48 hours to 7 days after onset. Thus, caution on using systemic fibrinolysis must be carefully considered to minimize morbidity and mortality. There are several absolute and relative contraindications that need to be assessed before administration (Table 1).

Using fibrinolytics as the main reperfusion therapy is recommended as soon as possible after the onset of the event. Infusion for up to 2 hours provokes fewer bleeding events than infusion for 24–48 hours. The preferred agents for systemic fibrinolysis are streptokinase and recombinant tissue plasminogen activator. Streptokinase is the oldest form of fibrinolytic agent that effectively dissolves clots in any vessel system, including pulmonary artery, coronary artery, deep vein, and cerebral vasculature. It is a polypeptide derived from beta-hemolytic Lancefield group C streptococci, which can turn plasminogen into proteolytic enzyme plasmin to lyse fibrin clots. Its half-life ranges between 23 to 29 minutes and resolves up to 48 hours in the plasma (Grierson and Bjornsson 1987). Recombinant tissue plasminogen activator is a synthetic form of tissue plasminogen activator that has undergone several biomodifications to improve efficacy and pharmacological properties. Their mechanism of action is the same as natural tissue plasminogen activator (e.g., streptokinase), but they cleave more specifically to Arg561-Val562 peptide bond to activate plasminogen into plasmin. Alteplase is one of the most widely used human plasminogen activators, while reteplase and tenecteplase are two of rtPA that possess a longer half-life than that of alteplase. All of them are administered intravenously to provide the systemic effect of thrombolysis. To reverse the effects of thrombolysis, the FDA has approved the usage of aminocaproic acid as an inhibitor (Bunc et al. 2020).

Surgical Embolectomy

Surgical embolectomy is an invasive procedure employing open thoracotomy for the direct extraction of thrombi in the pulmonary vasculature. At that time, successful embolectomy was achieved following the aid of a cardiopulmonary bypass machine due to that the procedure causes massive bleeding and solely yields grave prognosis during operation Currently, surgical embolectomy is indicated only for patients having contraindication to fibrinolytics, failed attempts of catheter-assisted embolectomy, or severe shock (which can cause rapid death). Furthermore, its anatomical indication includes large emboli occluding proximal pulmonary emboli (causing deep shock) (Agnelli and Becattini 2015).

Patients having acute PE indicated for surgery are immediately transferred into the operating room and placed in veno-arterial extracorporeal membrane oxygenation or rapid anesthetic induction with the placement of cardiopulmonary bypass. Placement of transoesophageal echocardiography gives information regarding intracardiac anatomy, right ventricle function, and chamber characteristics. Median sternotomy followed by incision on the pulmonary artery display visualization to the interior lumen of the artery. Desjardin gall stone forceps or Russian forceps are best used to carefully and gently remove the embolus from the lumen. Usage of Fogarty embolectomy catheter through the arteriotomy is considered an alternative If the thrombus has lodged distally in the vasculature, a classic incision of the left atrium is made, and a Foley catheter is then inserted into the orifice of the pulmonary vein. Bolus injection of saline dislodges the thrombi back to the proximal portion of the pulmonary artery, reached via pulmonary artery incision. Postoperative heparinization in the intensive care unit is commenced to anticipate recurrent embolism by maintaining a constant range of activated thromboplastin time of 60–80 seconds. Warfarin, a vitamin K antagonist, is administered to prevent subsequent formation of thrombus in any known underlying diseases for the next six months (Thaler, Pabinger, and Ay 2015).

Percutaneous Mechanical Thrombectomy

Percutaneous mechanical thrombectomy (PMT) involves the minimally invasive insertion of a catheter-based device to disintegrate and remove large emboli from the lumen. Mechanical thrombectomy is preferred for patients having contraindications to systemic fibrinolysis when rapid treatment could minimize the prognosis of massive acute PE. Ultrasound has been used in conjunction with the device to increase sensitivity localization of thrombus in the lumen. Furthermore, heparin is administered before the procedure to inhibit clot cascade during insertion of the device. Heparin or direct thrombin inhibitor (e.g., bivalirudin) is given initially, then an estimated 6 Fr guiding catheter is used to reach the location of thrombus intravenously. The guiding catheter could be crossed with a hydrophilic guidewire (Chan, Woods, and Shorr 2010).

This approach can use several different methods, such as thrombus fragmentation by rotating pigtail catheter, rheolytic and aspiration thrombectomy, and suction embolectomy. Table 2 summarizes the specific methods (Chan, Woods, and Shorr 2010).

Table 2. Summary of various methods of percutaneous mechanical thrombectomy

Methods	Processes
Thrombus Fragmentation	Using balloon angioplasty or rotating pigtail catheter to mechanically digest the thrombus (conventional) Using impeller to macerate thrombus No aspiration occurs.
Rheolytic and Aspiration Thrombectomy	Using a high-pressure saline jet or pulse-power spray of rtPA solution at the tip of the catheter to create a vacuum for fragmentation and aspiration.
Suction Embolectomy	Using combination method of mechanical thrombus fragmentation and rheolytic aspiration catheter technology to achieve thrombus removal.

Anticoagulant Therapy

Initial anticoagulation treatment of PE includes administration of conventional anticoagulants (e.g., unfractionated heparin [UFH] or low molecular weight heparin [LMWH]), thrombin inhibitors (e.g., rivaroxaban and apixaban), and anti-Xa inhibitor (e.g., dabigatran). Before the emergence of systemic fibrinolytic agents, heparin is known to be used as initial treatment for acute pulmonary embolism). Moreover, UFH is indicated to treat PE with hypotension or shock, instead of LMWH, fondaparinux, or direct oral anticoagulants, according to ESC guidelines (Konstantinides et al. 2020). Since recommended usage of fibrinolytic agents, sole anticoagulant therapy is best indicated for patients having a submassive PE (intermediate to low risk), due to its slower onset of action, or to be used on bottom administration of fibrinolytic agents in any acute settings. Quantifying the risk of 30-day mortality in acute pulmonary embolism could be done by utilizing the Simplified Pulmonary Embolism Severity Index (sPESI). High-risk pulmonary embolism includes one of the following characteristics, such as age older than 80 y.o., active cancer diagnosed within 12 months and or undergoing treatment, chronic cardiopulmonary diseases, heart rate > 100/min, systolic blood pressure < 100 mmHg, arterial blood oxygen saturation <90% with or without supplemental oxygen (Yamashita et al. 2020).

Follow-up treatment after initial management is required to stabilize patients; this should be regarded as a continuum of the holistic management of acute PE. According to the American College of Clinical Pharmacology guidelines (2012), anticoagulation must proceed with careful consideration for a minimum of three months for patients with venous thromboembolism, including acute PE, irrespective of underlying diseases. This recommendation persists if no transient risk factors occur, such as trauma, surgery, immobilization, pregnancy, or hormonal replacement therapy. Additionally, patients with low kidney functions are given unfractionated heparin only, whose elimination involves the reticuloendothelial system. Low molecular weight heparin and direct oral anticoagulants are cleared via kidney, explaining its cautious usage on patients with renal failure (Guyatt et al. 2012).

Venous Filters

A venous filter is a triangular-shaped metal stent used to entrap mobile thrombi throughout the venous system. Insertion of venous filter involves minimally invasive procedure using guidewire via the jugular vein Several indications of using venous filters are acute PE with contraindication to anticoagulation, prophylaxis in high-risk populations (e.g., cancer, immobilization), the emergence of deep vein thrombosis (DVT), or hemodynamic instability in patients. Venous filters are commonly utilized before the manipulation of deep vein clots using a catheter device to prevent subsequent adverse embolic events (White et al. 2000).

When the filters are clogged with mobile thrombi, patients experience several symptoms, such as bilateral/unilateral swollen legs (according to the position of the filter), leg pain, or sensations of internal pressure in the legs; these signs need to be evaluated for replacement of the filter. If the patient complains of severe pain in another area of the abdomen, chest, or neck, then the physician is urged to assess complications related to stent migration or vein perforation. Undersized filter or introduction of central line catheter are some of the causes Thus, immediate extraction of the dislodged filter is required to prevent fatal complications (White et al. 2000).

Method

Sources and Materials

This chapter on treatment updates for acute PE follows guidelines published by the European Society of Cardiology (ESC) and the American Heart

Association (AHA). Recommendations from both guidelines are compared to each other to provide deeper insight to the reader in terms of evidence level, strength, and relevancy to recent research. Methods used to gather reliable sources involved simple literature reviews with manual searches based on the aforementioned keywords in any search engine. To expand sensitivity and specificity during the searching process, Boolean operators were utilized in variance to keywords in the engine. Inclusion criteria were all accessible articles (except for clinical trials) and articles written in English. On the other hand, exclusion criteria comprised editorials, unpublished articles, news, and expert opinions.

Structures

This section conforms with the scientific principles of conducting a literature review, consisting of searching and evaluating literature, identifying problems, addressing methods, outlining structures, and organizing the writing. Sources are critically analyzed and evaluated to obtain relevant solutions to the problem mentioned in the introduction/background. This chapter used thematic analysis to ensure coverage of the large amounts of recent information regarding treatment updates for acute PE.

Results and Discussion

Guidelines are made to facilitate the decision-making of health professionals in everyday practice, thus they ought to be updated accordingly based on the constantly developing science of medicine. Critical evaluation ensures valid grading of strength and level of evidence, as well as assessment of risk-benefit dilemma in every recommendation.

Globally, treatment of acute PE follows guidelines published by the professional working research group of the ESC and/or advice vetted by the AHA. Both groups are involved in the extensive review of trials and research regarding the management of acute PE, providing insights and important points for effective diagnosis and prompt treatment of the disease. The ESC Committee for Practice Guidelines has actively revised the updated guidelines published in 2019 with additional reviews by experts in their field. The AHA does not publish updated guidelines regarding the management of acute PE in a single bundle; instead, it actively monitors the basic guidelines and incorporates separate publications in its journal. Consistently, the final document reflects consensus opinion throughout the entire committee. Reviewing recommendations from both guidelines may give a side-to-side comparison, expanding readers' point of view for its basic reasoning and terms of supporting evidence.

Table 3. Classification of recommendation and level of evidence

Recommendation Strength		Level of Evidence	
Class I [Benefit >>> risk]	Procedure/Treatment should be performed	Level A	Data/evidence derived from multiple randomized trials or meta-analyses
Class IIa [Benefit >> risk]	Procedure/Treatment is reasonable to be performed	Level B	Data/evidence derived from single randomized trials or large non-randomized studies
Class IIb [Benefit ≥ risk]	Procedure/Treatment may be considered to be performed	Level C	Data/evidence derived from retrospective studies, registry, small studies, or expert opinion
Class III [Benefit < risk]	Procedure/Treatment should not be performed		

Recommendations of Acute Treatment for Massive Pulmonary Embolism

Recommendation 1: Weight-Adjusted Bolus of Injected Unfractionated Heparin Should Be Initiated without Delay in Massive Acute Pulmonary Embolism

In the Multicentre Emergency Medicine Pulmonary Embolism in the Real-World Registry (EMPEROR) study, UFH was commonly used as a first-line agent to treat acute PE due to its fast onset of action, short half-life, and easy reversibility using antifibrinolytic regimens. Its usage reached up to 47.8% of patients suffering from acute PE, exceeding the combined numbers of patients treated with either fondaparinux or LMWH (Pollack et al. 2011). Biochemically, UFH binds to factor Xa and thrombin, inhibiting further cascade activation. Its anticoagulant activity heavily relies on equivalent inhibition of activated factor X and thrombin-activated conversion of fibrinogen to fibrin in the cascade sequence. The penta-saccharides unit in the UFH also blocks activation of factor IX and silence the forwarding effect of factor X activation. Its unpredictable pharmacokinetic profile explains its rapidly changing effect in the plasma due to binding to various endogenous proteins, including heparin-binding protein, histidine-rich glycoprotein, fibronectin, and von Willebrand factor (vWF) (Leentjens et al. 2017).

Table 4. Summary recommendation of acute treatment for massive pulmonary embolism

No	Recommendations	ESC 2019	AHA 2011
1.	A weight-adjusted bolus of injection unfractionated heparin (UFH) should be initiated without delay in massive PE	Class I*, level C**	Class I*, level A**
2.	Systemic fibrinolysis is recommended for massive PE	Class I*, level B**	Class IIa*, level B**
3.	Surgical pulmonary embolectomy is recommended for patients with massive PE, in whom fibrinolysis is contraindicated or has failed	Class I*, level C**	Class IIa*, level C**
4.	Percutaneous mechanical thrombectomy is recommended for patients with massive PE, in whom fibrinolysis is contraindicated or has failed	Class IIa*, level C**	
5.	Norepinephrine and/or dobutamine is recommended in patients with massive PE	Class IIa*, level C**	No recommendation
6.	Extracorporeal membrane oxygenation (ECMO) is recommended in combination with surgical embolectomy or percutaneous mechanical thrombectomy in massive PE and circulatory collapse	Class IIb*, level C**	No recommendation

*Class of recommendation
**Level of evidence

In terms of biological effects, UFH manifests higher efficacy in patients in comparison with other types of anticoagulants. In a previous meta-analysis, weight-adjusted LMWH exhibited a statistically nonsignificant lower rate of reperfusion in PE, compared with UFH (odds ratio, OR 0.63, 95% confidence interval, CI [0.33, 1.88]) (Agnelli and Becattini 2015). Further single randomized trials performed by Senturk et al. showed that the incidence of 30-day death was 8.2% or 17.3% in patients administered LMWH or UFH respectively ($p = 0.031$). Although the two treatments exhibited similar efficacy in terms of reducing all-cause mortality, lower bleeding tendency was observed in the LMWH group (Senturk et al. 2016). In determining whether LMWH is a better choice than UFH during the initial treatment of acute PE, low rate of creatinine clearance (< 30 ml/min/1.73m^2) is one of the factors considered. Due to various studies presenting controversial preferences for LMWH or UFH during the initial management of acute PE, the ESC 2019 guidelines conclude by announcing the level of evidence as C for this recommendation. In contrast, AHA 2011 recommends UFH administration without delay due to level A evidence corresponding to a randomized control trial (RCT) published in 1960 by Barritt and Jordan (Jaff et al. 2011). These results showed a reduced rate of mortality with heparin administration in acute PE patients, regardless of any side effects, although the effect was not statistically significant and the sample size was small (n = 35) (Fannin and Gray 1989). Thus, even though there are concerns regarding the potential side effects of heparin administration in patients with acute PE, most findings have suggested benefits to be gained from this recommendation.

Recommendation 2: Systemic Fibrinolysis Is Recommended for Massive Pulmonary Embolism

The rationale for PE patients being given fibrinolysis is to rapidly overcome the hemodynamic collapse and disrupted gas exchange due to pulmonary blood flow obstruction. Fibrinolysis would chemically break down the clotting complex into smaller subunits. Dissolution of the complex into D-dimer or other fibrin degradation products helps reduce clot size, which enables blood to flow through pulmonary arteries. It serves as a 'rapid start' in the reperfusion process compared to other given medications, such as anticoagulation. Its fast onset of action provides benefit to the ones suffering from massive pulmonary embolism, more against the risk of systemic bleeding (Piazza and Goldhaber 2010). According to a previous trial by Tibbutt et al., more evidence of thrombolysis was noted when patients with acute PE were treated with streptokinase (a fibrinolytic agent), compared with those treated with heparin alone. The reduction in systolic and mean pulmonary arterial pressure was significant in patients treated with streptokinase (Tibbutt et al. 1974). As massive PE confers such a high risk of mortality, direct fibrinolysis without early risk assessment is still beneficial; underlying this recommendation is the fact that bleeding risk assessment consumes considerable time, during which the condition of the patient may progressively worsen. Retrospectively analyzing the evidence, most of the trials were conducted before the 21st century. Few follow-up trials conducted with a similar method have resulted in the same conclusions as those of Tibbutt et al. Furthermore, switching to fibrinolytics occurred at the beginning of the 1980s due to the higher efficacy of these agents in treating acute PE, compared with the use of anticoagulants (such as heparin) alone (J.M. and M.A. 2017). According to AHA 2011 guidelines, fibrinolysis is best used in acute PE when bleeding events occur with intermediate-to-low risk. It is worth noting that before the 21st century, researchers investigating fibrinolytic agents placed more emphasis on the risk of bleeding events (and with hindsight may be considered to have been moderately biased in this respect). As the data obtained to make these recommendations predominantly came from several single trials carried out between the 1970s and the 1990s, it was not unreasonable for the AHA to propose class IIa and level B evidence for this recommendation in 2011 (Jaff et al. 2011). However, as more trials are being conducted, systemic fibrinolysis is currently the first-line treatment for acute PE in clinical settings, and therefore closer to the class I recommendation promoted by the ESC 2019 guidelines (Konstantinides et al. 2020).

Recommendation 3: Surgical Pulmonary Embolectomy Is Recommended for Patients with Massive PE, in Whom Fibrinolysis Is Contraindicated or Has Failed

Surgical pulmonary embolectomy involves the extraction of blood clots in the main pulmonary artery via open surgery. It results in a similar outcome to fibrinolysis but only affects locally. Massive pulmonary embolism requires immediate relief of the obstructions in the pulmonary trunks. Thus, surgical pulmonary embolectomy also serves as definitive treatment of massive PE for the ones who are contraindicated for systemic fibrinolysis.

Previous studies showed that other indications for this procedure are failure in response to fibrinolysis, cardiopulmonary arrest, interatrial septum defect, and the presence of clots in the right atrium (Azari, Bigdelu, and Moravvej 2015). A meta-analysis involving up to 1,300 participants in 46 studies discovered the linear association between mortality and prevalence of cardiopulmonary arrest before embolectomy. Thus, rapid initiation of surgical procedures in cases of massive PE prevents subsequent complications, as well as grave prognosis. Most studies have shown the benefits of surgical pulmonary embolectomy as an alternative therapeutic option to systemic fibrinolysis for massive PE with hemodynamic collapse; therefore, this is categorized as a minimum class IIa recommendation (Fukuda and Daitoku 2017).

In the middle of the 20th century, surgical embolectomy was only indicated for patients with refractory cardiogenic shock for whom there were no other therapeutic options. These actions manifested in a large number of perioperative deaths (up to 30%). Refinement of surgical procedures was subsequently carried out in a number of health centers, with outcomes beginning to improve (Poterucha et al. 2015). Case reports and series have been the predominant forms of evidence for surgical embolectomy until now, partly because usage has been restricted to patients suffering from massive cardiovascular collapse due to acute PE, where carrying out the surgical procedure has been perceived to bring more benefit than risk, compared with not treating at all. Thus, the evidence for this recommendation has been classified as level C. Surgical embolectomy is considered a class I recommendation in the ESC 2019 guidelines, while it is classified as class IIa in the AHA 2011 guidelines. Although both guidelines accepted level C evidence for this recommendation, differences in how the particular evidence was interpreted account for the distinctive class recommendations. AHA guidelines advise caution when considering major, invasive operations as they lean heavily on findings of case studies published in the 1990s; this point of view prioritizes a multidisciplinary view of benefits and risks when handling cases of massive PE (Jaff et al. 2011). However, the ESC 2019 recommendation is based solely on results published by Meneveau et al. from a prospective single-center registry study conducted in 1995 (which involved 488 patients); this showed that rescue surgical embolectomy led to better in-hospital prognosis for patients who did not respond to fibrinolysis (Meneveau et al. 2006). Further notes are written, albeit, that surgical embolectomy is still recommended when appropriate expertise and resources are available on-site (Konstantinides et al. 2020). Thus, this recommendation is better classified as class IIa.

Recommendation 4: Percutaneous Mechanical Thrombectomy Is Recommended for Patients with Massive PE, in Whom Fibrinolysis Is Contraindicated or Has Failed

Percutaneous mechanical thrombectomy (PMT) is still indicated for patients having failed to achieve therapeutic benefits or contraindication to systemic fibrinolysis. Studies conducted by Bunc et al. showed that 80% of patients with massive PE fully recovered following PMT intervention. Although this method uses a similar mechanism to surgical embolectomy for extracting clots, it relies on catheter devices inserted through the femoral or brachial vein and can also be used in combination with means of catheter-directed thrombolysis or pharmaco-mechanical thrombectomy.

Like surgery, PMT is best performed within 14 days of onset of the acute presentation. A previous case series showed a 100% success rate for PMT management in 20 patients with acute PE The previous case series exhibited a 100% success rate of PMT management in 20 patients with acute PE. Details of health parameters, such as pulmonary arterial pressure and oxygen saturation, improved significantly post PMT intervention with no recurrence of embolism during 16 months of follow-up (Dudzinski, Giri, and Rosenfield 2017; Liu et al. 2018). According to Toma et al., a retrospective analysis showed that aspiration thrombectomy using the FlowTriever thrombectomy system successfully removed lodged clots in 32 out of 34 patients with massive or high-risk submassive acute PE (one patient died during follow-up, with others showing decreased mean pulmonary artery pressure) (Toma et al.

2020). As PMT was found to be effective for managing massive acute PE, this study was then reconducted as a prospective FLARE-ED trial focusing on treating patients suffering from intermediate-risk or submassive acute PE with this minimally invasive procedure (Tu et al. 2019). Complications related to this procedure occur at a rate of up to 3.3%, such as rupture of veins, bleeding, or cardiopulmonary distress. Although complications may be imminent in rare cases, PMT is still considered for patients who have massive acute PE that has not been successfully treated by the use of systemic fibrinolysis (Vesely 2002). It is therefore reasonable for both guidelines to propose the same class IIa recommendation, with level C evidence determined from studies involving massive PE.

Recommendation 5: Norepinephrine And/or Dobutamine Is Recommended in Patients with Massive PE

Norepinephrine and dobutamine are intravenous drugs that could rapidly elevate cardiac output and give a vasoconstrictive effect. Norepinephrine binds to adrenergic receptor spread in the entire cardiovascular system, but it acts dominantly on alpha-1 subtype adrenergic receptor in arterial smooth muscle cells than the beta-1 subtype in cardiac myocytes. Thus, norepinephrine prominently manifests in systemic arterial vasoconstriction. It gives the extra benefit of increased perfusion pressure when administered during the early phase of shock (Hamzaoui, Scheeren, and Teboul 2017). On the other hand, dobutamine has two different stereoisomers in the prepared solution. One isomer acts as a strong alpha-1 agonist, while the other isomer has strong beta-1 and beta-2 agonistic properties, as well as alpha-1 antagonism. Due to the existence of two reciprocal alpha-1 effects, both isomers null the direct vascular effect but works predominantly on the effect of cardiac inotropism. Thus, dobutamine serves to increase cardiac output without affecting the vascular system (Dubin, Lattanzio, and Gatti 2017).

In ESC 2019 guideline, the proposed recommendation is solely based on findings of the case series in the year 1992. It stated that dobutamine improved oxygen transport and tissue oxygenation rate in patients having acute massive PE; however, it could not explain the reason behind the similar PaO_2 level despite administration of dobutamine. Besides, no study was cited by ESC 2019 focusing discussion on the utilization of norepinephrine to massive PE conditions (Manier and Castaing 1992). To conclude, this recommendation is considered prematurely classified with an insignificant level of evidence in the ESC 2019 guideline. No similar recommendation was proposed in AHA 2011 guideline (Jaff et al. 2011; Konstantinides et al. 2020).

Recommendation 6: Extracorporeal Membrane Oxygenation (ECMO) Is Recommended in Combination with Surgical Embolectomy or Percutaneous Mechanical Thrombectomy in Massive PE and Circulatory Collapse

During invasive operations in unstable patients, a valuable tool has been widely used to bypass blood out of patients' vascular systems to a blood-pumping machine. The remarkably progressed tool was more equipped nowadays than ever before. It is the extracorporeal membrane oxygenation (ECMO). ECMO possesses multi-functional features besides pumping blood with similar pressure from the heart, such as continuous oxygenation, waste particle filtration, and temperature controller. Its natural properties on becoming supportive therapy are the reason for its usage during invasive surgery, which significantly improved mortality rate over years (Makdisi and Wang 2015). ECMO, however, also has several intermediate-to-long term side effects, like increased bleeding rate in the first 90-day post ECMO, increased risk of stroke or thromboembolism, and postoperative infection (Zangrillo et al. 2013). In a multi-center series of 52 cases, usage of ECMO in patients who failed fibrinolysis is associated with a worse prognosis compared to ECMO performed in addition to surgical embolectomy. Massive PE patients who are solely supported with ECMO exhibit severe presentation. Thus, this finding suggested that ECMO would be better used to complement surgical embolectomy for patients with massive PE (Meneveau et al. 2018).

Recommendations of Acute Treatment for Submassive Pulmonary Embolism

Recommendation 1: Initiation of Anticoagulation Is Recommended without Delay in Patients with Submassive Acute Pulmonary Embolism

Anticoagulation is the primary therapy for patients with submassive acute PE whereas it offers inhibition of larger clot formation. Choice of anticoagulants differs from each facility, primarily consisting of heparin or direct oral anticoagulants (DOACs). In the EINSTEIN and AMPLIFY studies, early administration of LMWH helped to reduce the early risk of mortality during the first 48 hours (before switching to DOACs) (Nguyen et al. 2021). Recommendation of anticoagulation irrespective of type of PE stems from the fact that untreated acute PE is associated with a 25% risk of death, while initial anticoagulation minimizes the risk of death regardless of bleeding risk profile

(Leentjens et al. 2017). This rationale was confirmed by studies conducted in the 1960s that demonstrated the benefits of heparin in comparison to no treatment at all (Torbicki et al. 2008). Despite using references based on old evidence, numerous recent reports of submassive PE still follow this guideline recommendation, including cases of adolescent PE, submassive PE with syncope as initial symptoms, and elderly patients suffering from PE with comorbid (Lim, Roy, and Kevat 2021; Wang, Chen, and Di 2014; Clark et al. 2013).

Choice of anticoagulant depends on the respective clinical setting. Consistent results were found in a meta-analysis of 12 studies (n = 1951), where treatment of submassive PE with LMWH was associated with similar all-cause mortality (OR = 1.2; 95% CI [0.59-2.45]) and bleeding events (OR = 0.67; 95% CI [0.36-1.27]), compared to use of UFH (Jaff et al. 2011). Hence, anticoagulants seem to be the initial treatment of choice for suspected PE in most centers, gaining support from both guidelines as class I recommendation, despite the lack of stronger evidence.

Recommendation 2: Systemic Fibrinolysis Is Considered for Patients with Submassive PE Judged to Have Evidence of Hemodynamic Deterioration

Systemic fibrinolysis exhibits benefits for short-term treatment during the initial onset of acute pulmonary embolism. According to ESC/AHA recommendation, it is best suitable for patients presenting massive pulmonary embolism, except when there are absolute contraindications. Submassive pulmonary embolism manifests in right ventricular dysfunction or hypokinesia, yet it has a stable hemodynamic condition. Despite that, untreated submassive pulmonary embolism would rapidly deteriorate and result in cardiovascular collapse. Submassive PE judged for evidence of hemodynamic deterioration, such as signs of systemic shock, hypotension, tachycardia, fast/irregular breathing, or altered consciousness, are treated the same way as massive PE (Sekhri et al. 2012).

Systemic fibrinolysis provides rapid dissolution of clot obstructing major pulmonary vessels. Prospective cohort studies involving 86 patients with submassive PE showed that intravenous fibrinolysis reduced the rate of right ventricular dysfunction by up to 20%. Furthermore, pulmonary artery pressure during pre-and post-treatment decreased to 14 ± 3 mmHg (Rehman et al. 2020). The PEITHO (Pulmonary Embolism Thrombolysis) trial, which concluded at the end of 2014, compared groups treated with heparin only or tenecteplase plus heparin in 1,000 patients with submassive PE. The tenecteplase plus heparin group exhibited reduced cardiac deterioration and all-cause mortality, even though this combination caused an increase of 6.3% in the rate of major bleeding. This was reinforced by the 2016 American College of Chest Physicians guidelines, which recommended systemic fibrinolysis in cases of submassive PE with clinical decompensation or low bleeding risk profile (Rali and Criner 2018). These recent findings account for the fact that the ESC 2019 guidelines promoted the level of evidence to B for this recommendation. This precedent had not been set during the year that the AHA published its guidelines (2011), which merely utilized recent evidence or reports to support its recommendation. As administration of fibrinolytics may cause bleeding, it should be accompanied by a comprehensive assessment of an individual's bleeding profile. Nonetheless, the recommendation made by each guideline is based on their respective point of view regarding the condition of hemodynamic deterioration in submassive acute PE settings.

The ESC defines hemodynamic deterioration as any of the following clinical statuses: i) need of cardiopulmonary resuscitation; ii) systolic blood pressure < 90 mmHg or vasopressors needed to achieve > 90 mmHg blood pressure; iii) persistent systolic blood pressure < 90 mmHg lasting longer than 15 mins with no evidence of new-onset arrhythmia, sepsis, or hypovolemia (Konstantinides et al. 2020). On the other hand, the AHA defines hemodynamic deterioration as evidence of new hemodynamic instability, worsening respiratory insufficiency, severe right ventricular dysfunction confirmed with echocardio-graphy or CT scan, or myocardial infarct confirmed with elevated cardiac biomarkers. Evidence of hemodynamic deterioration confirmed by supportive examination without worsening clinical status is considered as indication for fibrinolysis in the AHA 2011 but not the ESC 2019 guidelines. Such discrepancies may underlie distinct class recommendations with respect to the administration of fibrinolysis for submassive PE judged to have hemodynamic deterioration.

Recommendation 3: Percutaneous Mechanical Thrombectomy or Surgical Embolectomy Are Not Recommended for Patients with Submassive PE with No Clinical Worsening

Based on AHA 2011 guidelines, this recommendation stems from case series suggesting a mortality rate between 20% and 30% during embolectomy operations (Stein et al. 2007). Another set of multicenter data analyzed by the Society of Thoracic Surgery Database revealed a rate of 12% in-hospital mortality, increasing to 32% when patients were submitted to surgical embolectomy (Keeling et al. 2016). Therefore, performing surgical embolectomy must involve careful pre-operative assessment as it provides the highest relative benefit for patients having a rapid onset of clinical worsening. Pre-operative assessment is also required with PMT, which can result in pulmonary hemorrhage or right chamber perforation due to puncture of major pulmonary arteries; the occurrence of perforation is rare but potentially serious (Biederer et al. 2006). Another retrospective report showed that 92% of submassive PE patients with clinical deterioration who were treated with PMT achieved technical success despite 8% major bleeding and 15% in-hospital deaths (Chechi et al. 2009). As the samples did not strongly represent patients who were stable, it is reasonable to weigh the risk of performing these invasive treatments to be higher than its benefit when administered to patients with hemodynamically stable submassive PE. Finally, low-level pieces of evidence from registries and pooled results of case series concluded in an evidence level of C for PMT or surgery in stable patients with submassive PE (Tafur et al. 2017).

Recommendation 4: LWMH or Fondaparinux Is Recommended over UFH in Submassive Acute Pulmonary Embolism Treated with Parenteral Anticoagulation

UFH exhibits a higher risk of bleeding which accounts for selective monitoring toward patients having submassive acute pulmonary embolism with bleeding risk. In the first 48 hours of administration, UFH fails to achieve therapeutic effect in terms of aPTT value measured from blood samples of patients with intermediate- to low-risk of PE, thus making UFH clinically difficult to maintain appropriate anticoagulation time frame for fast onset during its initial treatment. In a cohort study conducted by Cossette et al. involving 3,066 patients, UFH was shown to produce a 4.72-fold higher risk of bleeding (95% CI [2.17-10.30], $p < 0.001$), compared with LMWHs. However, this study did not specifically target patients with PE, which implied that the study merely described bleeding risk differences when using different kinds of available anticoagulants (Cossette et al. 2010).

Another interesting finding from an RCT revealed that overall, 3-month follow-up mortality was higher in patients given fondaparinux, compared with patients given UFH (5.2% vs. 4.4%, respectively), but the bleeding rate was lower (2% vs. 2.4% respectively). This finding positively correlates with the pharmacological properties of LMWHs, which specifically inhibit only factor Xa. Despite the aforementioned data, initial treatment with the two anticoagulants manifested different outcomes. Intravenous UFH exhibited a higher mortality rate, compared with subcutaneous fondaparinux (1.1% vs. 0.8%, respectively), similar to some of the findings published in the form of meta-analyses of multiple RCTs (Investigator 2003). At the end of follow-up, LMWHs produced a nonsignificant reduction in mortality rate, compared with UFH (Peto OR 0.84, 95% CI [0.7-1.01], p = 0.07) with less frequent major bleeding (Peto OR 0.69, 95% CI [0.5 – 0.95], p = 0.02).(Robertson and Jones 2017) Despite the fact that LMWHs and UFH have not been studied in the context of submassive PE populations in previous research, ESC 2019 guidelines recommend class I usage of LMWHs over UFH in these patients.

It is well known that initial anticoagulation is strongly suggested in all patients presenting various prognoses of acute PE in order to minimize mortality. Multidisciplinary discussion is required for delivering comprehensive decisions to give either anticoagulant to patients with submassive PE. AHA 2011 guidelines do not propose any recommendations for either anticoagulant, advising that choice should be based on clinical settings for individual patients (Jaff et al. 2011; Konstantinides et al. 2020). Thus, careful risk assessment to choose the appropriate anticoagulant is best performed for patients presenting submassive PE.

Recommendation 5: Systemic Fibrinolysis Is Not Recommended in Patients with Submassive PE

The mortality rate of submassive PE varies within individuals. According to a previous prospective cohort involving 209 hemodynamically stable patients, only 31% of cases of submassive PE exhibited right ventricular dysfunction confirmed by echocardiography with 5-10% of the cases developing progressive deterioration (Nguyen et al. 2021). In the I-COPER registry, the mortality rate reached 16.3% in patients having submassive PE with right ventricular hypokinesis. A 25% decreased rate of mortality was observed following fibrinolytic administration in this study. However, other registries, such as RIETE and EMPEROR, exhibited an increased 5-10% risk of death following the same treatment (Kucher et al. 2005; Jaff et al. 2011). Additionally, in the MAPPET-3 (Management Strategies and Prognosis of Pulmonary Embolism) trial, fibrinolysis reduced in-hospital mortality when submassive PE patients were given tissue plasminogen activator plus heparin compared to heparin alone (11% vs. 24.6%, p = 0.006). No fatal bleeding was observed in both groups (Konstantinides et al. 2002). That all these past trials accounted for the fact that administration of fibrinolytics may potentially reverse the clinical status of patients having submassive pulmonary embolism are indeed controversial until now. Based on these findings, AHA 2011 does not recommend routine usage of fibrinolytics in the settings of submassive PE.

In the PEITHO study, fibrinolysis demonstrated a significantly reduced risk of mortality (OR = 0.44; 95% CI 0.23-0.87; p = 0.02) in those patients who have worsening clinical status during the onset of submassive pulmonary embolism. Yet, the risk of major bleeding was increased up to 2.8 folds (OR = 2.8, 95%CI 1.00 – 7.86) (Rali and Criner 2018; Nguyen et al. 2021). ESC 2019 guideline established the statement based on findings published by PEITHO trial, which recommended careful decision on using fibrinolytics in submassive PE. Thus, it is reasonable that both guidelines proposed this recommendation as similar class III level B evidence. It does not strongly support routine fibrinolysis in submassive PE with no hemodynamic deterioration unless any bleeding profile is acceptable enough so that the benefit of fibrinolysis1w surpasses its risk of bleeding (Jaff et al. 2011; Konstantinides et al. 2020).

Table 5. Summary recommendation of acute treatment for submassive pulmonary embolism

No	Recommendations	ESC 2019	AHA 2011
1.	Initiation of anticoagulation is recommended without delay in patients with submassive acute pulmonary embolism	Class I*, level C**	
2.	Systemic fibrinolysis is considered for patients with submassive PE judged to have evidence of hemodynamic deterioration	Class I*, level B**	Class IIb*, level C**
3.	Percutaneous mechanical thrombectomy or surgical embolectomy are not recommended for patients with submassive PE with no clinical worsening	No recommendation	Class III*, level C**
4.	LWMH or fondaparinux is recommended over UFH in submassive acute pulmonary embolism treated with parenteral anticoagulation	Class I*, level A**	No recommendation
5.	Systemic fibrinolysis is not recommended in patients with submassive PE	Class III*, level B**	
6.	NOAC is recommended in preference to VKA in patients with submassive acute pulmonary embolism	Class I*, level A**	No recommendation
7.	NOAC is not recommended in patients with severe renal impairments, during pregnancy and lactation, and in patients with antiphospholipid syndrome	Class III*, level C**	No recommendation
8.	Therapeutic fixed-dose low molecular weight heparin (LMWH) based on early pregnancy body weight is recommended for pregnant women without hemodynamic instability	Class I*, level B**	No recommendation

*Class of recommendation; **Level of evidence

Recommendation 6: NOAC Is Recommended in Preference to VKA in Patients with Submassive Acute Pulmonary Embolism

Novel oral anticoagulants (NOAC) are synthetically made agents that directly inhibit both thrombin and factor Xa. Despite more specific pharmacodynamic action in the coagulation pathway than vitamin K antagonist (VKA), NOAC has been found to exhibit effective anticoagulation outcomes for patients with acute pulmonary embolism. In a randomized, double-blind study, a twice-daily dosage of 10 mg apixaban, one of the NOACs, was revealed to be non-inferior to VKA in terms of mortality when treating acute PE (HR 0.84, 95% CI 0.6 – 1.18) and exhibited lower risk of major bleeding (HR 0.31, 95% CI 0.17 – 0.55, $p < 0.001$) (Curto et al. 2013). Additionally, in another randomized trial, a twice-daily dosage of 15 mg rivaroxaban, another NOAC, also showed similar efficacy with the conventional VKA therapy (HR 0.9, 95% CI 0.76 – 1.07), as well as lower bleeding rate (HR 0.49, 95% CI 0.31 – 0.79, $p = 0.003$) (Bailey 2012). A recent finding by RE-COVER investigation emphasized that dabigatran, as one of the NOACs, has a similar effect on pulmonary embolism recurrent compared to VKA for treatment of acute PE (HR 1.09, 95%CI 0.76 – 1.57) (Schulman et al. 2014). Thus, better outcomes and less bleeding were found following treatment using NOAC than VKA. These discoveries have led to the amendment of ESC guidelines by adding a recommendation to use NOACs when there is no contraindication as an initial anticoagulation treatment for patients with submassive PE. Multiple randomized trials strongly supported this recommendation as level A evidence (Konstantinides et al. 2020).

Recommendation 7: NOAC Is Not Recommended in Patients with Severe Renal Impairments, during Pregnancy and Lactation, and in Patients with Antiphospholipid Syndrome

NOACs are metabolized and excreted partially in the kidney. Dabigatran is hydrolyzed by carboxylesterases to the active substance with bioavailability reaching up to 6.5% and a half-life lasting for 24 hours. In addition, apixaban has 50% bioavailability with peak concentration reached within 3-4 hours post-administration. Rivaroxaban is absorbed in the GI tract with 80-90% bioavailability, having a half-life of approximately 5-9 hours. All of them, albeit differences in pharmacokinetic characteristics, have the same excretion pathway predominantly via the kidneys. In rivaroxaban-treated patients, the use of standard-dose in patients with severe renal impairment (creatinine clearance < 15 ml/min) reflects overdose of the drugs and causes a higher risk of bleeding (HR 2.2, 95% CI 1.1 – 4.5) (Ingrasciotta et al. 2018). However, the impact of mild to moderate renal insufficiency (creatinine clearance > 30 ml/min) did not pose any significant side effects in terms of major bleeding when given standard dosage of NOACs (HR 0.93, 95% CI 0.7 – 1.16, p = 0.153) (Gui et al. 2019).

According to the Royal College of Obstetricians and Gynaecologist's recent guidelines, the use of NOACs are not recommended for women who are currently breastfeeding (Goecke, Voigt, and Rath 2020). A narrative review revealed that little excreted amounts of NOACs can be found in human breast milk with only apixaban having greater excretion than the maximum allowed range. Nevertheless, there has been a lack of evidence supporting this statement, which requires larger and more valid studies (Daei, Khalili, and Heidari 2021). Furthermore, summary product characteristics published by FDA have classified NOACs as category C, where toxic effects during pregnancy have been demonstrated in animal research. Considering this fact, it is better to switch to alternative anticoagulants when given to pregnant patients having an acute pulmonary embolism (Goecke, Voigt, and Rath 2020). Anti-phospholipid syndrome (APS) is an autoimmune disease that signifies the production of auto-antibodies attacking various phospholipids, including spectrum findings of anticardiolipin, anti-β2 glycoprotein, and lupus anticoagulant.

The risk of thrombosis varies by the clinical characteristics of each patient. Fluctuating speed of thrombosis inside APS patients' bodies may manifest in exacerbating components of venous thromboembolism, therefore requiring constant monitoring of INR value when treated with anticoagulant. Vitamin K antagonists have been the preferred drug of choice for APS patients. However, there has been recent evidence that some APS patients develop warfarin resistance with unstable anticoagulation quality. Thus, guidelines published by different organizations have detailed that warfarin or vitamin K antagonist should be used as the first choice of treatment, but NOACs should only be considered in patients with stable anticoagulation with NOACs, warfarin-resistance profile, unwilling to undergo INR monitoring, and contraindication to warfarin (Pastori et al. 2021). To conclude, patients with different clinical statuses should not be generalized as fully contraindicated to NOACs, as well as considering its various strength of the evidence supporting the data.

Recommendation 8: Therapeutic Fixed-Dose Low Molecular Weight Heparin (LMWH) Based on Early Pregnancy Body Weight Is Recommended for Pregnant Women without Hemodynamic Instability

Both AHA 2011 and ESC 2019 agreed that therapeutic dosage of anticoagulation should be initiated without delay in all patients with submassive pulmonary embolism (Jaff et al. 2011; Konstantinides et al. 2020). However, several anticoagulants are contraindicated for pregnant women as they have potentially teratogenic effects. Low molecular weight heparin (LMWHs) is one of the drugs tested as category B (no evidence of adverse effects on humans) in pregnancy by the US Food and Drug Administration (FDA) (Services 2016). Meta-analysis of 18 studies comprising of RCTs and cohorts suggested that anticoagulation is correlated to 1.4-1.9% of major bleeding with an estimated recurrent VTE of 1.97% during pregnancy (Rupasinghe et al. 2013).

A similar study focusing on reviewing the safety and efficacy of LWMHs for treatment of VTE in pregnancy was conducted by Greer et al. No maternal death was reported following usage of LMWHs in pregnant women. Recurrent VTE events occurred in 0.86% (95% CI 0.55-1.28%) of pregnancies with a 1.98% rate of major bleeding associated with primary obstetric causes. Almost 85.4% of live births were reported in pregnant women who received LMWHs (Greer and Nelson-Piercy 2005). Thus, LMWHs are safe and effective to be used to treat any emerging VTE in pregnancy. However, cautious utilization may prevent significant bleeding events during pregnancy.

Recommendations for Chronic Treatment and Prevention of Recurrence

Recommendation 1: IVC Filters Should Be Considered in Patients with Acute PE and Absolute Contraindications to Anticoagulation

Inferior vena cava (IVC) filters insertion functions to prevent migration of peripheral thrombus up to the level of pulmonary arteries, thus subsequently reducing the risk of developing acute pulmonary embolism. IVC filter is inserted via catheter-based device through the femoral vein, which renders minimally invasive outcome. Its indication is continuing to expand, but it still holds the same principle as the previous guidelines mentioned. Some classic indications of IVC insertion include contraindication to anticoagulation, complication of anticoagulation which requires cessation, or failure of anticoagulation to prevent the propagation of thrombus. Contraindications to anticoagulation are risk of bleeding, cerebral lesions, acute hemorrhagic stroke, severe hypertension, severe renal or hepatic dysfunction (Deyoung and Minocha 2016). Recent findings have suggested that emerging intraprocedural or postprocedural complications are grounds for re-evaluating indications of inferior vena cava (IVC) filters for PE patients; for example, 4%–11% chance of vascular complications, 1% chance of filter migration, and 1%–14% chance of filter malfunction may be considered as not being caused by human error. Furthermore, these may not include other much more severe errors, such as filter fracture or perforation of great veins by the filters (Grewal, Chamarthy, and Kalva 2016).

In the PREPIC2 trial, it was concluded that there was no reduced risk of acute PE related to lower vein thrombosis when performing combined IVC filter insertion and anticoagulation compared to anticoagulation alone (Partovi, Davidson, and Patel 2016). This confirmed the findings of a prior trial showing that using retrievable IVC filters did not reduce the risk of symptomatic recurrent PE in the first three months for patients who could be treated with anticoagulation (Mismetti et al. 2015). However, a published meta-analysis involving 11 primary studies suggested that IVC filter placement reduced the incidence of PE by up to 50% and the risk of recurrent DVT by 70%, although all-cause mortality did not significantly differ in patients with or without filter placement. Nonetheless, this meta-analysis retrieved only low-to-moderate quality RCTs and cohorts with findings that were substantially similar across a range of sensitivity analyses (Bikdeli et al. 2017).

As proposed by both guidelines, low-to-moderate quality evidence in these past primary studies involving IVC filters signifies level C evidence. However, despite the level C evidence, recently updated findings regarding potential complications resulting from IVC placement prompted a change in the ESC 2019 recommendation to class IIa, providing additional insight into the different class of recommendation published in the AHA 2011 guidelines. To conclude, IVC filters provide optimal benefits only for PE patients with contraindication or failed use of anticoagulation as they could pose a risk of complications during or after the procedures.

Recommendation 2: IVC Filters Should Be Considered in Cases of PE Recurrence Despite Anticoagulation

The current consensus regarding the use of IVC filters to prevent cases of recurrent PE is somewhat unclear. In a study presented by Stein et al., a retrospective analysis showed that IVC filter placement was associated with reduced risk of death in unstable patients with PE across age groups. (Stein et al. 2007) This finding was also supported by the PREPIC trial, where IVC filters prevented recurrent PE ($p = 0.03$), despite more DVT occurrences (20.8% with filters vs. 11.6% without filters, $p = 0.02$). (Decousus 2005) Conversely, results of a population-based retrospective analysis of around 65,000 linked hospital discharge abstracts were negative overall with respect to the use of IVC filters. Insertion of IVC filters was not associated with reduced risk of rehospitalization for PE, despite usage in patients who initially manifested PE; this indicated the importance of future prospective studies to confirm the efficacy level of IVC filters among patients with recurrent PE.

With respect to filter placement, patients and physicians should be aware of the increased risk for venous thrombosis, ranging from 1.14- to 2.62-fold (White et al. 2000). In several case reports, a number of patients with hypercoagulable states, such as those suffering from antiphospholipid syndrome, died from massive PE following IVC filter placement; the reports described emboli stemming from organized thrombus formation proximally along the filter (Cherian and Gertner 2005).

To conclude, no stronger form of evidence (such as RCTs) has mentioned the benefits of IVC filters in preventing recurrence of PE; this reinforces the claim from both guidelines that this recommendation is classified as level C strength, with careful consideration of the balance between preventing the emergence of recurrent PE and thrombus formation in deep veins.

Recommendation 3: Patients with Submassive Pulmonary Embolism Are Carefully Considered for Discharge with Proper Anticoagulant Treatment during Outpatient Care

An RCT conducted in 2011 involved 344 patients with low-risk submassive PE equally divided into two treatment groups. Results revealed that 0.6% of outpatients developed recurrent PE within three months, whereas this was not the case for inpatients ($p = 0.011$). Additionally, 1.8% of outpatients suffered from major bleeding, whereas the inpatient group was not affected ($p = 0.086$) (Aujesky et al. 2011). However, other prospective multicenter studies showed that outpatient treatment of submassive PE with NT pro-BNP level < 500

pg/mL appeared to be safe, with no recorded deaths during the first 10 days or serious adverse events during a 3-month follow-up.(Agterof et al. 2010) In another study, 6 out of 297 patients had recurrent VTE (2%), while 3 of out 297 patients died during the 3-month follow-up (1%) with two major bleeding events (0.7%). Outpatient groups were selected based on predefined criteria, such as no hemodynamic instability, no active pain, no history of diseases or comorbidities, more than 3-month life expectancy, and not pregnant (Zondag et al. 2011).

Similar results were presented by Barco et al. in his team's prospective clinical investigation involving 525 patients treated with rivaroxaban with a 3-month outpatient follow-up; rates of major bleeding and non-fatal PEs were 1.2% and 0.6%, respectively, during the follow-up period. (Barco et al. 2020) Repeated studies with the aforementioned exclusion criteria for out-patient treatment indicated a similar risk of bleeding, deaths, and recurrent PE events. Considering the strength and validity of past data, the evidence is classified as level A. This therefore supports the notion that early discharge for outpatient treatment has to be carefully considered by physicians in order to ensure minimal risk of mortality and morbidity, as well as to increase the efficiency of treatment cost.

Table 6. Summary recommendation of chronic treatment and prevention of recurrence

No	Recommendations	ESC 2019	AHA 2011
1.	IVC filters should be considered in patients with acute PE and absolute contraindications to anticoagulation	Class IIa*, level C**	Class I*, level C**
2.	IVC filters should be considered in cases of PE recurrence despite anticoagulation	Class IIa*, level C**	
3.	Patients with submassive pulmonary embolism are carefully considered for discharge with proper anticoagulant treatment during outpatient care	Class IIa*, level A**	No recommendation
4.	Discontinuation of therapeutic oral anticoagulation after 3 m.o. in patients with first PE secondary to reversible risk factors	Class I*, level B**	Class I*, level A**
5.	Therapeutic anticoagulation for more than 3 m.o. is recommended for all patients with PE	Class I*, level A**	No recommendation
6.	In patients who are unable to take any form of oral anticoagulants, aspirin may be considered for extended VTE prophylaxis	Class IIb*, level B**	No recommendation
7.	Routine clinical evaluation of patients 3 – 6 m.o. after acute pulmonary embolism episode is recommended	Class I*, level B**	Class I*, level A**

*Class of recommendation; **Level of evidence

Recommendation 4: Discontinuation of Therapeutic Oral Anticoagulation after 3 Months. in Patients with First PE Secondary to Reversible Risk Factors

Oral anticoagulation provides specific protection against populations with high-risk factors of venous thromboembolism recurrence, such as D-dimer level higher than 250 mcg/l, obesity, elderly, male sex, or other post-thrombotic signs. As long as PE patients persistently have those risk factors, indefinite anticoagulation is essential. Previous studies showed that these populations would have the risk of recurrent venous thromboembolism (VTE) up to 10% in the first year, followed by 5% per year. Nevertheless, the population with transient risk factors would be at 1% risk of suffering from recurrent VTE in the first year, followed by 0.5% per year (Kearon et al. 2016). For patients with 8-10% cumulative risk of recurrent VTE in the first year, these populations experienced a greater chance of residual pulmonary vascular obstruction at 6 months. Therefore, extending anticoagulation beyond initial acute PE treatment minimizes similar events in near future. In a systematic review involving a total of 2387 patients from multiple studies, there were 96 recurrent VTEs occurred during the first 12 months after stopping anticoagulant therapy provoked by any transient risk factors. The annualized event rate was 3.1% per patient year (Singh et al. 2009). The risk was low enough to be justified by the task force, who recommended only 3 months of anticoagulant treatment regardless of the severity provoked by the aforementioned risk factors. This was due to several findings which could not establish the association between the severity of acute PE with that of the next recurrent event (Slabbynck, Clukers, and Galdermans 2020). It is assumed to exhibit little benefit from 6-month anticoagulation, when compared to only 3-month anticoagulation, for patients with unknown or transient risk factors. Extending the duration of anticoagulation for these populations may be considered against the increasing risk of bleeding events (Campbell et al. 2007). Based on both ESC 2019 and AHA 2011 guidelines, it is an absolute recommendation to give anticoagulation therapy for all acute PE patients for the first 3 months.

Recommendation 5: Therapeutic Anticoagulation for more than 3 Months is Recommended for All Patients with PE

According to findings in the previous recommendation, it is confirmed that the risk of recurrence of ceasing anticoagulants after 3 months follow up would be doubled when there are permanent risk factors, which will be further doubled during the next 18 months (Baglin et al. 2003). Despite that, a meta-analysis found out that 3 months of anticoagulant treatment resulted in a similar risk of recurrence compared to a longer duration of treatment in PE patients provoked by temporary risk factors. This recommendation stemmed from the fact that the risk of recurrent venous thromboembolism during 2 years is 1.5-fold higher in the less-than-3-month anticoagulation group (HR 1.52, 95% CI 1.14 – 2.02, p = 0.008).

This analysis was obtained in combined patient settings with and without temporary risk factors (Boutitie et al. 2011). Thus, it is necessary to provide an adequate period of 3-month anticoagulation regardless of the various presentation of acute PE.

Recommendation 6: In Patients Who Are Unable to Take Any Form of Oral Anticoagulants, Aspirin May Be Considered for Extended VTE Prophylaxis

Oral anticoagulants are contraindicated for some patients with bleeding risk after careful assessment. This recommendation serves to acknowledge alternatives to oral anticoagulants that could minimize the recurrent event of pulmonary embolism in patients indicated for indefinite anticoagulation, whilst preventing major bleeding. These are patients with first unprovoked episodes of acute pulmonary embolism, including the absence of any transient risk factors. In the studies, almost all patients were required to finish their 3-month anticoagulation treatment based on the class I recommendation. Then, they were randomized into two groups that would be followed up to 4 years. One group received a placebo tablet daily, and the other one received 100 mg aspirin daily. Both groups manifest a similar risk of recurrent venous thromboembolism (HR 0.74, 95% CI 0.52 – 1.05, p = 0.09) but significantly less major bleeding event happened in the aspirin group (HR 0.67, 95% CI 0.49 – 0.91, p = 0.01) (Brighton et al. 2012).

These results were different from the ones conducted in WARFASA (Warfarin and Aspirin) trial in 2012. There was a significant decrease of recurrent venous thromboembolism in the group who received aspirin 100 mg daily compared to the placebo group during two-year follow up (HR 0.58, 95% CI 0.36 – 0.93, p = 0.02), yet both groups had similar bleeding risk (p = 0.97) and deaths (p = 0.95) (Cecilia Becattini, M.D., Ph.D., Giancarlo Agnelli, M.D., Alessandro Schenone, M.D., Sabine Eichinger, Eugenio Bucherini, M.D., Mauro Silingardi, M.D., Marina Bianchi, M.D., Marco Moia, M.D., Walter Ageno, and Maria Rita Vandelli, M.D., Elvira Grandone, M.D., and Paolo Prandoni, M.D. 2012). To further confirm the fact, a recently published systematic review and meta-analysis of large 13 RCTs was conducted to assess the effectiveness of aspirin as alternative prophylaxis to prevent recurrent venous thromboembolism. Of the meta-analysis, the relative risk of venous thromboembolism given by aspirin did not significantly differ from that given by LMWHs (RR 0.76, 95% CI 0.37 – 1.56) and rivaroxaban (RR 1.52, 95% CI 0.56 – 4.12). The risk of adverse events, including major bleeding, also was not statistically significantly different in groups receiving aspirin versus other anticoagulants (Matharu et al. 2020). Thus, aspirin is not inferior to other anticoagulants when used as an alternative thromboprophylaxis treatment. ESC 2019 did not incorporate recently published meta-analyses into their discussion; therefore, it had not updated its recommendation strength level.

Considering the most recent research, the class IIb recommendation was not clinically relevant when oral anticoagulants are contraindicated for patients having venous thrombo-embolism (Konstan-tinides et al. 2020). Hence, clarity in determining class recommendation should be addressed in the future.

Recommendation 7: Routine Clinical Evaluation of Patients 3–6 Months after Acute Pulmonary Embolism Episode Is Recommended

Based on a multi-center prospective cohort conducted by FOCUS (Follow-up After Acute Pulmonary Embolism), the overall quality of life in 620 patients was scaled using EuroQoL Group 5-Dimension 5-Level Utility Index improved from 3 to 12 months since the onset of initial pulmonary embolism. Nonetheless, several independent factors which were associated with lower QoL and slower recovery of QoL were identified, such as female sex, history of cardiopulmonary diseases, older age, and previous VTE. First follow-up evaluation at 3 months represents a critical decision regarding the duration of anticoagulation or possible testing for any late residual PE (Valerio et al. 2021). Routine clinical evaluations at the first 3-month are meant to monitor lab bleeding profile during primary anticoagulation.

As per the previous recommendation, the second 3-month since the onset of acute PE represents detection of any residual late PE that could occur regardless of risk factors. Therefore, the course of evaluation is promptly based on the clinical characteristics of each patient (Ortel et al. 2020).

Conclusion

Both ESC 2019 and AHA 2011 guidelines are sufficient to support each other in terms of general treatment for acute PE. Some recommendations have not been updated, which is possibly counterproductive for the most recent published findings; these findings are generally measured as non-major recommendations with weak level of evidence. Several recommendations may not explicitly be proposed in both guidelines, which could be due to different timelines of evidence used by each recommendation. Hence, physicians should prioritize the best clinical judgment for every patient suffering from acute PE, while using these recommendations as general guidelines.

References

Agnelli, Giancarlo, and Cecilia Becattini. 2015. "Anticoagulant Treatment for Acute Pulmonary Embolism: A Pathophysiology-Based Clinical Approach." *European Respiratory Journal*, 45 (4): 1142–49. https://doi.org/10.1183/09031936.00164714.

Agterof, M. J., R. E.G. Schutgens, R. J. Snijder, G. Epping, H. G. Peltenburg, E. F.M. Posthuma, J. A. Hardeman, et al. 2010. "Out of Hospital Treatment of Acute Pulmonary Embolism in Patients with a Low NT-ProBNP Level." *Journal of Thrombosis and Haemostasis*, 8 (6): 1235–41. https://doi.org/10.1111/j.1538-7836.2010.03831.x.

Aujesky, Drahomir, Pierre Marie Roy, Franck Verschuren, Marc Righini, Joseph Osterwalder, Michael Egloff, Bertrand Renaud, et al. 2011. "Outpatient versus Inpatient Treatment for Patients with Acute Pulmonary Embolism: An International, Open-Label, Randomised, Non-Inferiority Trial." *The Lancet*, 378 (9785): 41–48. https://doi.org/10.1016/S0140-6736(11)60824-6.

Azari, Ali, Leila Bigdelu, and Zahra Moravvej. 2015. "Surgical Embolectomy in the Management of Massive and Sub-Massive Pulmonary Embolism: The Results of 30 Consecutive Ill Patients." *ARYA Atherosclerosis*, 11 (3).

Baglin, Trevor, Roger Luddington, Karen Brown, and Caroline Baglin. 2003. "Incidence of Recurrent Venous Thromboembolism in Relation to Clinical and Thrombophilic Risk Factors: Prospective Cohort Study." *Lancet*, 362 (9383): 523–26. https://doi.org/10.1016/S0140-6736(03)14111-6.

Bailey, Alison L. 2012. "Oral Rivaroxaban for the Treatment of Symptomatic Pulmonary Embolism." *Cardiology Review*, 28 (3): 1287–97. https://doi.org/10.1056/nejmoa1113572.

Barco, Stefano, Irene Schmidtmann, Walter Ageno, Rupert M. Bauersachs, Cecilia Becattini, Enrico Bernardi, Jan Beyer-Westendorf, et al. 2020. "Early Discharge and Home Treatment of Patients with Low-Risk Pulmonary Embolism with the Oral Factor Xa Inhibitor Rivaroxaban: An International Multicentre Single-Arm Clinical

Trial." *European Heart Journal*, 41 (4): 509–18. https://doi.org/10.1093/eurheartj/ehz367.

Belicová, Margita, V. Jankovičová, M. Ochodnický, and M. Mokáň. 2018. "Pulmonary Embolism." *Cardiology Letters* 27 (4): 204–11. https://doi.org/10.1084/jem.26.3. 387.

Biederer, Jürgen, Nikolas Charalambous, Friedrich Paulsen, Martin Heller, and Stefan Müller-Hülsbeck. 2006. "Treatment of Acute Pulmonary Embolism: Local Effects of Three Hydrodynamic Thrombectomy Devices in an Ex Vivo Porcine Model." *Journal of Endovascular Therapy*, 13 (4): 549–60. https://doi.org/10.1583/06-1862.1.

Bikdeli, Behnood, Saurav Chatterjee, Nihar R. Desai, Ajay J. Kirtane, Mayur M. Desai, Michael B. Bracken, Frederick A. Spencer, Manuel Monreal, Samuel Z. Goldhaber, and Harlan M. Krumholz. 2017. "Inferior Vena Cava Filters to Prevent Pulmonary Embolism: Systematic Review and Meta-Analysis." *Journal of the American College of Cardiology*, 70 (13): 1587–97. https://doi.org/10.1016/j.jacc.2017.07.775.

Boutitie, Florent, Laurent Pinede, Sam Schulman, Giancarlo Agnelli, Gary Raskob, Jim Julian, Jack Hirsh, and Clive Kearon. 2011. "Influence of Preceding Length of Anticoagulant Treatment and Initial Presentation of Venous Thromboembolism on Risk of Recurrence after Stopping Treatment: Analysis of Individual Participants' Data from Seven Trials." *Bmj*, 342 (7810): 1–9. https://doi.org/10.1136/bmj.d3036.

Brass, Lawrence F., Maurizio Tomaiuolo, John Welsh, Izmarie Poventud-Fuentes, Li Zhu, Scott L. Diamond, and Timothy J. Stalker. 2019. *Hemostatic Thrombus Formation in Flowing Blood. Platelets*. 4th ed. Elsevier Inc. https://doi.org/10.1016/B978-0-12-813456-6.00020-5.

Brighton, Timothy A., John W. Eikelboom, Kristy Mann, Rebecca Mister, Alexander Gallus, Paul Ockelford, Harry Gibbs, et al. 2012. "Low-Dose Aspirin for Preventing Recurrent Venous Thromboembolism." *New England Journal of Medicine*, 367 (21): 1979–87. https://doi.org/10.1056/nejmoa1210384.

Bunc, Matjaz, Klemen Steblovnik, Simona Zorman, and Peter Popovic. 2020. "Percutaneous Mechanical Thrombectomy in Patients with High-Risk Pulmonary Embolism and Contraindications for Thrombolytic Therapy." *Radiology and Oncology*, 54 (1): 62–67. https://doi.org/10.2478/raon-2020-0006.

Campbell, I. A., D. P. Bentley, R. J. Prescott, P. A. Routledge, H. G.M. Shetty, and I. J. Williamson. 2007. "Anticoagulation for Three versus Six Months in Patients with Deep Vein Thrombosis or Pulmonary Embolism, or Both: Randomised Trial." *British Medical Journal*, 334 (7595): 674–77. https://doi.org/10.1136/bmj.39098.583356.55.

Cecilia Becattini, M.D., Ph.D., Giancarlo Agnelli, M.D., Alessandro Schenone, M.D., Sabine Eichinger, M.D., M.D. Eugenio Bucherini, M.D., Mauro Silingardi, M.D., Marina Bianchi, M.D., Marco Moia, M.D., Walter Ageno, and Ph.D Maria Rita Vandelli, M.D., Elvira Grandone, M.D., and Paolo Prandoni, M.D. 2012. "Aspirin for Preventing the Recurrence of Venous Thromboembolism." *New England Journal of Medicine*, 366: 1959–67.

Center for Drug Evaluation and Research. 2016. "Immunogenicity- Related Considerations for Low Molecular Weight Heparin Guidance for Industry Immunogenicity- Related Considerations for Low Molecular Weight Heparin Guidance for Industry," *FDA, Guidance Document, February 2016*.

Ceresetto, J.M., and Marques M.A. 2017. "Systemic Fibrinolytic Therapy in Pulmonary Thromboembolism." *Jornal Vascular Brasileiro*, 16 (2): 119–27. http://www.embase.com/search/results?subaction=viewrecord&from=export&id=L617650286%0Ahttp://dx.doi.org/10.1590/1677-5449.007316.

Chan, C. M., C. Woods, and A. F. Shorr. 2010. "The Validation and Reproducibility of the Pulmonary Embolism Severity Index." *Journal of Thrombosis and Haemostasis*, 8 (7): 1509–14. https://doi.org/10.1111/j.1538-7836.2010.03888.x.

Chechi, Tania, Sabine Vecchio, Gaia Spaziani, Gabriele Giuliani, Federica Giannotti, Chiara Arcangeli, Andrea Rubboli, and Massimo Margheri. 2009. "Rheolytic Thrombectomy in Patients with Massive and Submassive Acute Pulmonary Embolism." *Catheterization and Cardiovascular Interventions*, 73 (4): 506–13. https://doi.org/10.1002/ccd.21858.

Cherian, Joseph, and Elie Gertner. 2005. "Recurrent Pulmonary Embolism despite Inferior Vena Cava Filter Placement in Patients with the Antiphospholipid Syndrome." *Journal of Clinical Rheumatology*, 11 (1): 56–58. https://doi.org/10.1097/01.rhu.0000152150.01274.1b.

Clark, Donald, David C. McGiffin, Louis J. Dell'Italia, and Mustafa I. Ahmed. 2013. "Submassive Pulmonary Embolism Where's the Tipping Point?" *Circulation*, 127 (24): 2458–64. https://doi.org/10.1161/CIRCULATIONAHA.112.000859.

Cossette, B., M. É Pelletier, N. Carrier, M. Turgeon, C. Leclair, P. Charron, D. Echenberg, T. Fayad, and P. Farand. 2010. "Evaluation of Bleeding Risk in Patients Exposed to Therapeutic Unfractionated or Low-Molecular-Weight Heparin: A Cohort Study in the Context of a Quality Improvement Initiative." *Annals of Pharmacotherapy*, 44 (6): 994–1002. https://doi.org/10.1345/aph.1M615.

Curto, Madelyn, Alexander S Gallus, Margot Johnson, Urszula Masiukiewicz, Raphael Pak, D Ph, John Thompson, et al. 2013. "Oral Apixaban for the Treatment of Acute Venous Thromboembolism." *Zeitschrift Fur Gefassmedizin*, 10 (3): 25–26. https://doi.org/10.1056/nejmoa1302507.

Daei, Maryam, Hossein Khalili, and Zinat Heidari. 2021. "Direct Oral Anticoagulant Safety during Breastfeeding: A Narrative Review." *European Journal of Clinical Pharmacology*, 77 (10): 1465–71. https://doi.org/10.1007/s00228-021-03154-5.

Decousus, Hervé. 2005. "Eight-Year Follow-up of Patients with Permanent Vena Cava Filters in the Prevention of Pulmonary Embolism: The PREPIC (Prévention Du Risque d'Embolie Pulmonaire Par Interruption Cave) Randomized Study." *Circulation*, 112 (3): 416–22. https://doi.org/10.1161/CIRCULATIONAHA.104.512834.

Deyoung, Elliot, and Jeet Minocha. 2016. "Inferior Vena Cava Filters: Guidelines, Best Practice, and Expanding Indications." *Seminars in Interventional Radiology*, 33 (2): 65–70. https://doi.org/10.1055/s-0036-1581088.

Diamond, Scott L. 2016. "Systems Analysis of Thrombus Formation." *Circulation Research*, 118 (9): 1348–62. https://doi.org/10.1161/CIRCRESAHA.115.306824.

Dubin, Arnaldo, Bernardo Lattanzio, and Luis Gatti. 2017. "The Spectrum of Cardiovascular Effects of Dobutamine - from Healthy Subjects to Septic Shock Patients." *Revista Brasileira de Terapia Intensiva*, 29 (4): 490–98. https://doi.org/10.5935/0103-507X.20170068.

Dudzinski, David M., Jay Giri, and Kenneth Rosenfield. 2017. "Interventional Treatment of Pulmonary Embolism." *Circulation: Cardiovascular Interventions*, 10 (2): 1–10. https://doi.org/10.1161/CIRCINTERVENTIONS.116.004345.

Fannin, T. F., and W. J. Gray. 1989. "Anticoagulant Drugs in the Eldery." *British Medical Journal*, 298 (6667): 184. https://doi.org/10.1136/bmj.298.6667.184.

Fukuda, Ikuo, and Kazuyuki Daitoku. 2017. "Surgical Embolectomy for Acute Pulmonary Thromboembolism." *Annals of Vascular Diseases*, 10 (2): 107–14. https://doi.org/10.3400/avd.ra.17-00038.

Giordano, Nicholas J., Paul S. Jansson, Michael N. Young, Kaitlin A. Hagan, and Christopher Kabrhel. 2017. "Epidemiology, Pathophysiology, Stratification, and Natural History of Pulmonary Embolism." *Techniques in Vascular and Interventional Radiology*, 20 (3): 135–40. https://doi.org/10.1053/j.tvir.2017.07.002.

Goecke, Tamme, Franziska Voigt, and Werner Rath. 2020. "Reducing the Risk of Venous Thromboembolism during Pregnancy and the Puerperium." *Journal of Maternal-Fetal and Neonatal Medicine*, 33 (14): 2359–65. https://doi.org/10.1080/14767058.2018.1550064.

Greer, Ian A., and Catherine Nelson-Piercy. 2005. "Low-Molecular-Weight Heparins for Thromboprophylaxis and Treatment of Venous Thromboembolism in Pregnancy: A Systematic Review of Safety and Efficacy." *Blood*, 106 (2): 401–7. https://doi.org/10.1182/blood-2005-02-0626.

Grewal, Simer, Murthy R. Chamarthy, and Sanjeeva P. Kalva. 2016. "Complications of Inferior Vena Cava Filters." *Cardiovascular Diagnosis and Therapy*, 6 (6): 632–41. https://doi.org/10.21037/cdt.2016.09.08.

Grierson, David S., and Thorir D. Bjornsson. 1987. "Pharmacokinetics of Streptokinase in Patients Based on Amidolytic Activator Complex Activity." *Clinical Pharmacology and Therapeutics*, 41 (3): 304–13. https://doi.org/10.1038/clpt.1987.32.

Gui, Yi Yue, Song Zou, Wen Long Yang, Shen Zhen Gong, Zhi Fu Cen, Zhong Hui Xie, and Kai Jun Cui. 2019. "The Impact of Renal Function on Efficacy and Safety of New Oral Anticoagulant in Atrial Fibrillation Patients: A Systemic Review and Meta-Analysis." *Medicine (United States)*, 98 (48). https://doi.org/10.1097/MD.0000000000018205.

Guyatt, Gordon H., Elie A. Akl, Mark Crowther, David D. Gutterman, and Holger J. Schünemann. 2012. "Executive Summary: Antithrombotic Therapy and Prevention of Thrombosis, 9th Ed: American College of Chest Physicians Evidence-Based Clinical Practice Guidelines." *Chest*, 141 (2 SUPPL.): 7S-47S. https://doi.org/10.1378/chest.1412S3.

Hamzaoui, Olfa, Thomas W.L. Scheeren, and Jean Louis Teboul. 2017. "Norepinephrine in Septic Shock: When and How Much?" *Current Opinion in Critical Care*, 23 (4): 342–47. https://doi.org/10.1097/MCC.0000000000000418.

Ingrasciotta, Ylenia, Salvatore Crisafulli, Valeria Pizzimenti, Ilaria Marcianò, Anna Mancuso, Giuseppe Andò, Salvatore Corrao, Piera Capranzano, and Gianluca Trifirò. 2018. "Pharmacokinetics of New Oral Anticoagulants: Implications for Use in Routine Care." *Expert Opinion on Drug Metabolism and Toxicology*, 14 (10): 1057–69. https://doi.org/10.1080/17425255.2018.1530213.

Investigator, Matisse. 2003. "Subcutaneous Fondaparinux versus Intravenous Unfractionated Heparin in the Initial Treatment of Pulmonary Embolism." *New England Journal of Medicine*, no. 349: 1695–1792.

Jaff, Michael R., M. Sean McMurtry, Stephen L. Archer, Mary Cushman, Neil Goldenberg, Samuel Z. Goldhaber, J. Stephen Jenkins, et al. 2011. "Management of Massive and Submassive Pulmonary Embolism, Iliofemoral Deep Vein Thrombosis, and Chronic Thromboembolic Pulmonary Hypertension: A Scientific Statement from the American Heart Association." *Circulation*, 123 (16): 1788–1830. https://doi.org/10.1161/CIR.0b013e318214914f.

Kearon, Clive, Elie A. Akl, Joseph Ornelas, Allen Blaivas, David Jimenez, Henri Bounameaux, Menno Huisman, et al. 2016. "Antithrombotic Therapy for VTE Disease: CHEST Guideline and Expert Panel Report." *Chest*, 149 (2): 315–52. https://doi.org/10.1016/j.chest.2015.11.026.

Keeling, W. Brent, Thor Sundt, Marzia Leacche, Yutaka Okita, Jose Binongo, Yi Lasajanak, Lishan Aklog, and Omar M. Lattouf. 2016. "Outcomes After Surgical Pulmonary Embolectomy for Acute Pulmonary Embolus: A Multi-Institutional Study." *Annals of Thoracic Surgery*, 102 (5): 1498–1502. https://doi.org/10.1016/j.athoracsur.2016.05.004.

Konstantinides, Stavros, Annette Geibel, Gerhard Heusel, Fritz Heinrich, and Wolfgang Kasper. 2002. "Heparin plus Alteplase Compared with Heparin Alone in Patients with Submassive Pulmonary Embolism." *New England Journal of Medicine*, 347 (15): 1143–50. https://doi.org/10.1056/nejmoa021274.

Konstantinides, Stavros V., Guy Meyer, Héctor Bueno, Nazzareno Galié, J. Simon R. Gibbs, Walter Ageno, Stefan Agewall, et al. 2020. "2019 ESC Guidelines for the Diagnosis and Management of Acute Pulmonary Embolism Developed in Collaboration with the European Respiratory Society (ERS)." *European Heart Journal*, 41 (4): 543–603. https://doi.org/10.1093/eurheartj/ehz405.

Kucher, Nils, Elisa Rossi, Marisa De Rosa, and Samuel Z. Goldhaber. 2005. "Prognostic Role of Echocardiography among Patients with Acute Pulmonary Embolism and a Systolic Arterial Pressure of 90 Mm Hg or Higher." *Archives of Internal Medicine*, 165 (15): 1777–81. https://doi.org/10.1001/archinte.165.15.1777.

Laurentius, Andrea, and Rina Ariani. 2020. "Diagnostic Comparison of Anterior Leads T-Wave Inversion and McGinn-White Sign in Suspected Acute Pulmonary Embolism: A Systematic Review and Meta-Analysis." *Hong Kong Journal of Emergency Medicine*. https://doi.org/10.1177/1024907920966520.

Leentjens, Jenneke, Mike Peters, Anne C. Esselink, Yvo Smulders, and Cornelis Kramers. 2017. "Initial Anticoagulation in Patients with Pulmonary Embolism: Thrombolysis, Unfractionated Heparin, LMWH, Fondaparinux, or DOACs?" *British Journal of Clinical Pharmacology*, 83 (11): 2356–66. https://doi.org/10.1111/bcp.13340.

Lim, Adeline Yi Ling, John Roy, and Ajay Kevat. 2021. "Management of Submassive Bilateral Pulmonary Embolism in an Adolescent Female." *Case Reports in Pulmonology*, 2021. https://doi.org/10.1155/2021/1678528.

Liu, Bing, Ming Yuan Liu, Li Hong Yan, Jun Wei Yan, Jiang Wu, Xue Fei Jiao, and Ming Jin Guo. 2018. "Percutaneous Mechanical Thrombectomy Combined with Catheter-Directed Thrombolysis in the Treatment of Acute Pulmonary Embolism and Lower Extremity Deep Venous Thrombosis: A Novel One-Stop Endovascular Strategy."

Journal of International Medical Research, 46 (2): 836–51. https://doi.org/10.1177/0300060517729898.

Mackman, Nigel. 2012. "New Insights into the Mechanisms of Venous Thrombosis." *Journal of Clinical Investigation*, 122 (7): 2331–36. https://doi.org/10.1172/JCI60229.

Makdisi, George, and I. Wen Wang. 2015. "Extra Corporeal Membrane Oxygenation (ECMO) Review of a Lifesaving Technology." *Journal of Thoracic Disease*, 7 (7): E166–76. https://doi.org/10.3978/j.issn.2072-1439.2015.07.17.

Manier, G., and Y. Castaing. 1992. "Influence of Cardiac Output on Oxygen Exchange in Acute Pulmonary Embolism." *American Review of Respiratory Disease*, 145 (1): 130–36. https://doi.org/10.1164/ajrccm/145.1.130.

Mata, Robin, Gabrielle McDermott, and Lorenzo Diaz. 2020. "Massive Pulmonary Embolism as a Cause of Cardiac Arrest: Navigating Unknowns in Life After Death." *Cureus*, 12 (5). https://doi.org/10.7759/cureus.8361.

Matharu, Gulraj S., Setor K. Kunutsor, Andrew Judge, Ashley W. Blom, and Michael R. Whitehouse. 2020. "Clinical Effectiveness and Safety of Aspirin for Venous Thromboembolism Prophylaxis after Total Hip and Knee Replacement: A Systematic Review and Meta-Analysis of Randomized Clinical Trials." *JAMA Internal Medicine*, 180 (3): 376–84. https://doi.org/10.1001/ jamainternmed.2019.6108.

Meneveau, Nicolas, Benoit Guillon, Benjamin Planquette, Gaël Piton, Antoine Kimmoun, Lucie Gaide-Chevronnay, Nadia Aissaoui, et al. 2018. "Outcomes after Extracorporeal Membrane Oxygenation for the Treatment of High-Risk Pulmonary Embolism: A Multicentre Series of 52 Cases." *European Heart Journal*, 39 (47): 4196–4204. https://doi.org/10.1093/eurheartj/ehy464.

Meneveau, Nicolas, Marie France Séronde, Marie Cécile Blonde, Pierre Legalery, Katy Didier-Petit, Florent Briand, Fiona Caulfield, François Schiele, Yvette Bernard, and Jean Pierre Bassand. 2006. "Management of Unsuccessful Thrombolysis in Acute Massive Pulmonary Embolism." *Chest*, 129 (4): 1043–50. https://doi.org/10.1378/chest.129.4.1043.

Mismetti, Patrick, Silvy Laporte, Olivier Pellerin, Pierre Vladimir Ennezat, Francis Couturaud, Antoine Elias, Nicolas Falvo, et al. 2015. "Effect of a Retrievable Inferior Vena Cava Filter plus Anticoagulation vs Anticoagulation Alone on Risk of Recurrent Pulmonary Embolism: A Randomized Clinical Trial." *JAMA - Journal of the American Medical Association*, 313 (16): 1627–35. https://doi.org/10.1001/jama.2015.3780.

Nguyen, Phillip C., Hannah Stevens, Karlheinz Peter, and James D. McFadyen. 2021. "Submassive Pulmonary Embolism: Current Perspectives and Future Directions." *Journal of Clinical Medicine*, 10 (15). https://doi.org/10.3390/jcm10153383.

Ortel, Thomas L., Ignacio Neumann, Walter Ageno, Rebecca Beyth, Nathan P. Clark, Adam Cuker, Barbara A. Hutten, et al. 2020. "American Society of Hematology 2020 Guidelines for Management of Venous Thromboembolism: Treatment of Deep Vein Thrombosis and Pulmonary Embolism." *Blood Advances*, 4 (19): 4693–4738. https://doi.org/10.1182/bloodadvances.2020001830.

Partovi, Sasan, Jon C. Davidson, and Indravadan J. Patel. 2016. "Implications and Limitations of the PREPIC2 Study-the Interventionist's Perspective." *Cardiovascular Diagnosis and Therapy*, 6 (3): 259–61. https://doi.org/10.21037/ cdt.2016.01.03.

Pastori, Daniele, Danilo Menichelli, Vittoria Cammisotto, and Pasquale Pignatelli. 2021. "Use of Direct Oral Anticoagulants in Patients With Antiphospholipid Syndrome: A Systematic Review and Comparison of the International Guidelines." *Frontiers in Cardiovascular Medicine*, 8 (August). https://doi.org/10.3389/fcvm.2021.715878.

Piazza, Gregory, and Samuel Z. Goldhaber. 2010. "Fibrinolysis for Acute Pulmonary Embolism." *Vascular Medicine*, 15 (5): 419–28. https://doi.org/10.1177/1358863X 10380304.

Pollack, Charles V., Donald Schreiber, Samuel Z. Goldhaber, David Slattery, John Fanikos, Brian J. O'Neil, James R. Thompson, et al. 2011. "Clinical Characteristics, Management, and Outcomes of Patients Diagnosed with Acute Pulmonary Embolism in the Emergency Department: Initial Report of EMPEROR (Multicenter Emergency Medicine Pulmonary Embolism in the Real World Registry)." *Journal of the American College of Cardiology*, 57 (6): 700–706. https://doi.org/10.1016/ j.jacc.2010.05.071.

Poterucha, Timothy J., Brian Bergmark, Sary Aranki, Tsuyoshi Kaneko, and Gregory Piazza. 2015. "Surgical Pulmonary Embolectomy." *Circulation*, 132 (12): 1146–51. https://doi.org/10.1161/CIRCULATIONAHA.115.015916.

Rali, Parth M., and Gerard J. Criner. 2018. "Submassive Pulmonary Embolism." *American Journal of Respiratory and Critical Care Medicine*, 198 (5): 588–98. https://doi.org/ 10.1164/rccm.201711-2302CI.

Rehman, Nadeem U., Mohd Iqbal Dar, Manish Bansal, and R. R. Kasliwal. 2020. "Clinical Outcomes of Submassive Pulmonary Embolism Thrombolysis—an Indian Experience." *Egyptian Heart Journal*, 72 (1). https://doi.org/10.1186/s43044-020-00123-8.

Riedel, Martin. 2001. "Acute Pulmonary Embolism 2: Treatment." *Heart* 85 (3): 351–60. https://doi.org/10.1136/heart.85.3.351.

Robertson, Lindsay, and Lauren E. Jones. 2017. "Fixed Dose Subcutaneous Low Molecular Weight Heparins versus Adjusted Dose Unfractionated Heparin for the Initial Treatment of Venous Thromboembolism." *Cochrane Database of Systematic Reviews*, 2017 (2). https://doi.org/10.1002/14651858.CD001100.pub4.

Rupasinghe, M., T. C. Hollenbeck, S. Guzman-Reyes, M. M. Shetty, A. Giezentanner, D. Cattano, and E. G. Pivalizza. 2013. "Anticoagulant Therapy for Venous Thrombo-embolism during Pregnancy: A Systematic Review and a Meta-Analysis of the Literature: A Rebuttal." *Journal of Thrombosis and Haemostasis*, 11 (4): 787–88. https://doi.org/10.1111/jth.12135.

Saxena, Pankaj, Hassiba Smail, and David C. McGiffin. 2016. "Surgical Techniques of Pulmonary Embolectomy for Acute Pulmonary Embolism." *Operative Techniques in Thoracic and Cardiovascular Surgery*, 21 (2): 80–88. https://doi.org/10.1053/j.optech stcvs.2017.02.001.

Schulman, Sam, Ajay K. Kakkar, Samuel Z. Goldhaber, Sebastian Schellong, Henry Eriksson, Patrick Mismetti, Anita Vedel Christiansen, et al. 2014. "Treatment of Acute Venous Thromboembolism with Dabigatran or Warfarin and Pooled Analysis."

Circulation, 129 (7): 764–72. https://doi.org/10.1161/CIRCULATIONAHA.113.004450.

Sekhri, Vishal, Nimeshkumar Mehta, Naveen Rawat, Stuart G. Lehrman, and Wilbert S. Aronow. 2012. "Management of Massive and Nonmassive Pulmonary Embolism." *Archives of Medical Science*, 8 (6): 957–69. https://doi.org/10.5114/aoms.2012.32402.

Senturk, Aysegul, Elif Yilmazel Ucar, Serdar Berk, Tevfik Ozlu, Bulent Altlnsoy, Gul Dabak, Ebru Caklr, Esra Ekbic Kadloglu, Hadice Selimoglu Sen, and Savas Ozsu. 2016. "Should Low-Molecular-Weight Heparin Be Preferred over Unfractionated Heparin after Thrombolysis for Severity Pulmonary Embolism?" *Clinical and Applied Thrombosis/Hemostasis*, 22 (4): 395–99. https://doi.org/10.1177/1076029614564863.

Sharifi, Mohsen, Curt Bay, Sasan Nowroozi, Suzanne Bentz, Gayle Valeros, and Sara Memari. 2013. "Catheter-Directed Thrombolysis with Argatroban and TPA for Massive Iliac and Femoropopliteal Vein Thrombosis." *CardioVascular and Interventional Radiology*, 36 (6): 1586–90. https://doi.org/10.1007/s00270-013-0569-3.

Singh, Hardeep, Shrinidi Mani, Donna Espadas, Nancy Petersen, Veronica Franklin, and Laura A. Petersen. 2009. "Prescription Errors and Outcomes Related to Inconsistent Information Transmitted through Computerized Order Entry: A Prospective Study." *Archives of Internal Medicine*, 169 (10): 982–89. https://doi.org/10.1001/archinternmed.2009.102.

Slabbynck, Hans, Johan Clukers, and Daniella Galdermans. 2020. " Should oral anticoagulation be discontinued after 3 months in the setting of a first high-risk pulmonary embolism secondary to a major transient/reversible risk factor?" *European Respiratory Journal*. https://doi.org/10.1183/13993003.02028-2019.

Stein, Paul D., Majd Alnas, Afzal Beemath, and Nikunj R. Patel. 2007. "Outcome of Pulmonary Embolectomy." *American Journal of Cardiology*, 99 (3): 421–23. https://doi.org/10.1016/j.amjcard.2006.08.050.

Tafur, Alfonso J., Fadi E. Shamoun, Salma I. Patel, Denisse Tafur, Fabiola Donna, and M. Hassan Murad. 2017. "Catheter-Directed Treatment of Pulmonary Embolism: A Systematic Review and Meta-Analysis of Modern Literature." *Clinical and Applied Thrombosis/Hemostasis*, 23 (7): 821–29. https://doi.org/10.1177/1076029616661414.

Thaler, Johannes, Ingrid Pabinger, and Cihan Ay. 2015. "Anticoagulant Treatment of Deep Vein Thrombosis and Pulmonary Embolism: The Present State of the Art." *Frontiers in Cardiovascular Medicine*, 2 (July): 1–7. https://doi.org/10.3389/ fcvm.2015.00030.

Tibbutt, D. A., G. De J. Lee, A. A. Sharp, J. A. Davies, T. M. Holt, E. W.L. Fletcher, J. Hamill, M. Lea Thomas, and J. A. Anderson. 1974. "Comparison by Controlled Clinical Trial of Streptokinase and Heparin in Treatment of Life-Threatening Pulmonary Embolism." *British Medical Journal*, 1 (5904): 343–47. https://doi.org/10.1136/bmj.1.5904.343.

Toma, Catalin, Sameer Khandhar, Adrian M. Zalewski, Stephen J. D'Auria, Thomas M. Tu, and Wissam A. Jaber. 2020. "Percutaneous Thrombectomy in Patients with Massive and Very High-Risk Submassive Acute Pulmonary Embolism." *Catheterization and Cardiovascular Interventions*, 96 (7): 1465–70. https://doi.org/10.1002/ccd.29246.

Torbicki, Adam, Arnaud Perrier, Stavros Konstantinides, Giancarlo Agnelli, Nazzareno Galiè, Piotr Pruszczyk, Frank Bengel, et al. 2008. "Guidelines on the Diagnosis and Management of Acute Pulmonary Embolism." *European Heart Journal*, 29 (18): 2276–2315. https://doi.org/10.1093/eurheartj/ehn310.

Tu, Thomas, Catalin Toma, Victor F. Tapson, Christopher Adams, Wissam A. Jaber, Mitchell Silver, Sameer Khandhar, et al. 2019. "A Prospective, Single-Arm, Multicenter Trial of Catheter-Directed Mechanical Thrombectomy for Intermediate-Risk Acute Pulmonary Embolism: The FLARE Study." *JACC: Cardiovascular Interventions*, 12 (9): 859–69. https://doi.org/10.1016/j.jcin.2018.12.022.

Turetz, Meredith, Andrew T. Sideris, Oren A. Friedman, Nidhi Triphathi, and James M. Horowitz. 2018. "Epidemiology, Pathophysiology, and Natural History of Pulmonary Embolism." *Seminars in Interventional Radiology* 35 (2): 92–98. https://doi.org/10.1055/s-0038-1642036.

Ucar, Elif Yilmazel. 2019. "Update on Thrombolytic Therapy in Acute Pulmonary Thromboembolism." *Eurasian Journal of Medicine*, 51 (2): 185–89. https://doi.org/10.5152/eurasianjmed.2019.19291.

Valerio, Luca, Stefano Barco, Marius Jankowski, Stephan Rosenkranz, Mareike Lankeit, Matthias Held, Felix Gerhardt, et al. 2021. "Quality of Life 3 and 12 Months Following Acute Pulmonary Embolism: Analysis From a Prospective Multicenter Cohort Study." *Chest*, 159 (6): 2428–38. https://doi.org/10.1016/j.chest.2021.01.071.

Vesely, Thomas M. 2002. "Complications Related to Percutaneous Thrombectomy of Hemodialysis Grafts." *Journal of Vascular Access*, 3 (2): 49–57. https://doi.org/10.1177/112972980200300202.

Wang, Sheng Yu, Hui Chen, and Li Gai Di. 2014. "Caution for Acute Submassive Pulmonary Embolism with Syncope as Initial Symptom: A Case Report." *Journal of Thoracic Disease*, 6 (10): E212–16. https://doi.org/10.3978/j.issn.2072-1439.2014.08.11.

White, Richard H., Hong Zhou, Jinwoo Kim, and Patrick S. Romano. 2000. "A Population-Based Study of the Effectiveness of Inferior Vena Cava Filter Use among Patients with Venous Thromboembolism." *Archives of Internal Medicine*, 160 (13): 2033–41. https://doi.org/10.1001/archinte.160.13.2033.

Yamashita, Yugo, Takeshi Morimoto, Hidewo Amano, Toru Takase, Seiichi Hiramori, Kitae Kim, Maki Oi, et al. 2020. "Validation of Simplified PESI Score for Identification of Low-Risk Patients with Pulmonary Embolism: From the COMMAND VTE Registry." *European Heart Journal: Acute Cardiovascular Care*, 9 (4): 262–70. https://doi.org/10.1177/2048872618799993.

Zangrillo, Alberto, Giovanni Landoni, Giuseppe Biondi-Zoccai, Massimiliano Greco, Teresa Greco, Giacomo Frati, Nicolò Patroniti, Massimo Antonelli, Antonio Pesenti, and Federico Pappalardo. 2013. "A Meta-Analysis of Complications and Mortality of Extracorporeal Membrane Oxygenation." *Critical Care and Resuscitation*, 15 (3): 172–78.

Zondag, Wendy, I. C.M. Mos, D. Creemers-Schild, A. D.M. Hoogerbrugge, O. M. Dekkers, J. Dolsma, M. Eijsvogel, et al. 2011. "Outpatient Treatment in Patients with Acute Pulmonary Embolism: The Hestia Study." *Journal of Thrombosis and Haemostasis*, 9 (8): 1500–1507. https://doi.org/10.1111/j.1538-7836.2011.04388.x.

Biographical Sketches

Andrea Laurentius, MD

Affiliation: Faculty of Medicine Universitas Indonesia

Education: Medicine

Business Address: 06 Salemba St., Senen, Central Jakarta, Indonesia 10430

Research and Professional Experience:

- Associate Editor in J-AMSA International 2019/2020
- Scientific Secretariat of 31st Annual Scientific Meeting of Indonesian Heart Association 2022
- Follow up Coordinator for ArCoV Vaccine Clinical Research 2022
- Research Assistant on the Survey of Clinical Research Professionals for Competency by National Center for Global Health and Medicine (NCGM) 2022

Honors:

- Universitas Indonesia Rectorate Awardee for Outstanding Achievements 2019

Publications from the Last 3 Years:

Evaluation of Right Ventricular Outflow Tract Stenting as Palliative Treatment in Severely Cyanotic Tetralogy of Fallot: A Systematic Review and Meta-analysis of Observational Studies (*Journal of Tehran University Heart Center*, 2021, Vol 16, Issue 4).

Efficacy and Safety of Chrono-Modulated Statin Therapy as Modified Method of Treatment of Hypercholesterolemia (*World Heart Journal*, 2021, Vol 13, Issue 1).

Clinical Outcome of Renin-Angiotensin-Aldosterone System Blockers Treatment of Hypertensive Patients with COVID-19: A Systematic Review and Meta-Analysis (*Egyptian Heart Journal*, 2020).

Safety and Feasibility of Intracardiac Echocardiography in Comparison to Transoesophageal Echocardiography-Guided Percutaneous Interatrial Septum Defect Closure: A Systematic Review (*World Heart Journal*, 2020, Vol. 12, Issue 3).

Diagnostic comparison of anterior leads T-wave inversion and McGinn-White sign in suspected acute pulmonary embolism: A systematic review and meta-analysis (*Hong Kong Journal of Emergency Medicine*, 2020).

Moira Setiawan, MD

Affiliation: Faculty of Medicine, Universitas Indonesia

Education: Medicine

Business Address: 06 Salemba St., Senen, Central Jakarta, Indonesia 10430

Publications from the Last 3 Years:

A Comparative Effectiveness Systematic Review and Meta-analysis of Drugs for the Prophylaxis of Junctional Ectopic Tachycardia. *Curr Cardiol Rev.*, 2022;18(1).

Application of Transthoracic and Transesophageal Echocardiography in Guiding Patent Ductus Arteriosus Closure: An Evidence-Based Case Report and Systematic Review. *World Heart Journal*, 2021; 13(2).

Incidence Of Infective Endocarditis In Unrepaired Small Ventricular Septal Defect: A Systematic Review.

Pharmacology Management In Improving Exercise Capacity Of Patients With Fontan Circulation: A Systematic Review And Meta-Analysis. *Curr Cardiol Rev.*, 2022;18(5):34-49.

Kelvin Kohar, MD

Affiliation: Faculty of Medicine, Universitas Indonesia

Education: Medicine

Business Address: 06 Salemba St., Senen, Central Jakarta, Indonesia 10430

Publications from the Last 3 Years:

Comparison between the world health organization (WHO) and international society of hypertension (ISH) guidelines for hypertension. *Ann Med.*, 2022 Dec;54(1):837-84

Aditya Parawangsa, MD

Affiliation: Faculty of Medicine, Universitas Indonesia

Education: Medicine

Business Address: 06 Salemba St., Senen, Central Jakarta, Indonesia 10430

Eric Ferdinand, MD

Affiliation: Faculty of Medicine, Universitas Indonesia

Education: Medicine

Business Address: 06 Salemba St., Senen, Central Jakarta, Indonesia 10430

Publications from the Last 3 Years:

Application of Transthoracic and Transesophageal Echocardiography in Guiding Patent Ductus Arteriosus Closure: An Evidence-Based Case Report and Systematic Review. *World Heart Journal*, 2021; 13(2).

Chapter 2

Dual-Energy CT Performance in Pulmonary Embolism: A Systematic Review

Elvira Ruiz Castellano[1,2]
and Antonio Jesús Láinez Ramos-Bossini, MD[1,2,3]
[1]Department of Radiology,
Hospital Universitario Virgen de las Nieves,
Granada, Spain
[2] Biosanitary Research Institute, Granada, Spain
[3]Department of Psychiatry, School of Medicine,
University of Granada, Granada, Spain

Abstract

Computed tomography pulmonary angiography (CTPA) is the imaging technique of choice for the diagnosis of pulmonary embolism (PE). In clinical practice, multidetector single-energy CT (SECT) is the most commonly used worldwide. Dual-energy computed tomography (DECT) is a novel technology increasingly used in clinical practice. DECT offers different imaging postprocessing techniques based on the advantages of dual energy acquisition (e.g., linear blending, iodine maps, and virtual monoenergetic reconstructions) which maximize differences in contrast attenuation of tissues. This can aid in the diagnosis of PE. In this chapter, we report an up-to-date review of current evidence on the efficacy and possible advantages of DECT in the diagnosis of PE. We conducted a systematic review following the PRISMA guidelines. We performed structures searches in the main medical databases (PubMed, Web of Science, Scopus, Cochrane). We included observational studies, trials and systematic reviews analyzing the effectiveness of DECT in PE detection, contrast material used, and ionizing radiation rates. Our results indicate that DECT and SECT yield similar sensitivity and specificity

In: Understanding and Treating Acute Pulmonary Embolism
Editor: James K. Edwards
ISBN: 979-8-88697-149-1

values regarding PE detection. DECT allows the administration of a lower volume of iodine contrast agents and implies lower ionizing radiation. However, further studies are required to determine its cost-effectiveness compared to DECT.

Keywords: pulmonary embolism, computed tomography, dual-energy, diagnosis

Introduction

Venous thromboembolic disease (VTE), comprising deep vein thrombosis (DVT) and acute pulmonary embolism (PE), is a relatively common cardiovascular condition in the population, following myocardial infarction and stroke [1]. VTE occurs with an incidence of approximately 5% during and causes a very high morbidity and mortality, with PE generating the greatest impact and being the most difficult to diagnose [2].

The most common origin of PE is thought to be DVT, frequently in the lower limbs, with subsequent embolization to the pulmonary arteries. Although there is no consensus on the actual incidence of PE, some studies estimate it to be 39-115 per 100,000 persons, increasing with age, and in general terms it is slightly more frequent in men than in women (58 vs. 48 per 100,000 persons). However, the risk in women increases considerably with age due to hormonal factors (>500 per 100,000 people over 75 years) [1-3]. PE is traditionally considered an underdiagnosed disease, since it presents very non-specific symptoms and signs, and only a high degree of suspicion and the performance of imaging techniques, particularly computed tomography angiography of pulmonary arteries (CTPA), allow its diagnosis. Early diagnosis of this entity is important in order to initiate early treatment with anticoagulation, fibrinolysis, mechanical thrombectomy, or other medical/interventional treatments, which reduce the high mortality rate that accompanies it [1, 4, 5].

Over the years, awareness of PE underdiagnosis, its nonspecific clinical presentation, and the generalized increase in imaging tests have led to a marked increase in the detection of PE. Nevertheless, the mortality attributable to PE is high and difficult to estimate, since many causes of sudden cardiac death are thought to be secondary to PE. Thus, although this mortality seems to have decreased significantly in recent years, it has not decreased in parallel with the increase in PE detection [6].

The first step is to detect PE in patients lies in screening them according to Clinical Probability Scores (CPS) such as the Wells Score (WS) or the revised Geneva Scale (GS), and their simplified versions (WSs and GSs, respectively). These scores will help to take the second step, i.e., the decision to request the value of serum D-Dimer and/or CTPA [7]. The diagnostic algorithm ends up in ruling out PE or ordering a CTPA, either because the patient has a high probability according to any validated CPS or because the serum D-dimer is high. Interestingly, a low application of CPS in the management of PE at emergency departments (EDs) has been reported, with variable adherence depending on the age of the patient, the score used and the age adjustment of D-Dimer. This low adherence to the use of CPS has been reported to be associated with overuse of radiological examinations [8-11].

Once the high-risk patient has been selected, CTPA is considered the imaging technique of choice for the diagnosis of PE (class I recommendation) [1, 12]. Ventilation/perfusion (V/Q) scintigraphy, ventilation/perfusion single-photon emission computed tomography (V/Q SPECT), echocardiography, and magnetic resonance imaging (MRI) also play an important role in certain clinical situations [13]. Currently, CTPA includes two main subtypes. On the one hand, single-energy multidetector CT (SECT), is the most widely used in clinical practice worldwide, with a sensitivity of 83% and specificity of 96% in the diagnosis of acute PE [14]. On the other hand, dual-energy multidetector CT (DECT) is a new technology progressively replacing SECT for this purpose. Thanks to the high spatial resolution and isotropy of current multidetector CT machines, it is possible to diagnose even very small distal emboli [15]. Moreover, by means of different post-processing techniques using dual energy, DECT maximizes the differences in the attenuation spectrum of iodinated contrast, and even reduce the effective ionizing radiation dose administered to the patient. Despite the potential advantages of DECT over SECT, the recentness of the former and the small number of comparative studies between both techniques prevent definitive conclusions from being drawn. The aim of this chapter is to analyze the efficacy and possible advantages of DECT in the diagnosis of PE.

Methods

Eligibility Criteria

The design of this review and the selection criteria were based on the PICO search strategy. The population chosen was patients symptomatic or susceptible to PE; the intervention was DECT; the comparison was SECT; and the outcome was a diagnosis of PE. The Preferred Reporting Items for Systematic Reviews and Meta-Analyses (PRISMA) guidelines were followed [16]. Accordingly, the inclusion criteria were the following: published RCTs, meta-analysis, and systematic reviews on DECTs fundamentals, performance in pulmonary embolism, and comparing to SECT. The exclusion criteria were studies with quasi-experimental designs, letters, abstracts, or conference proceedings.

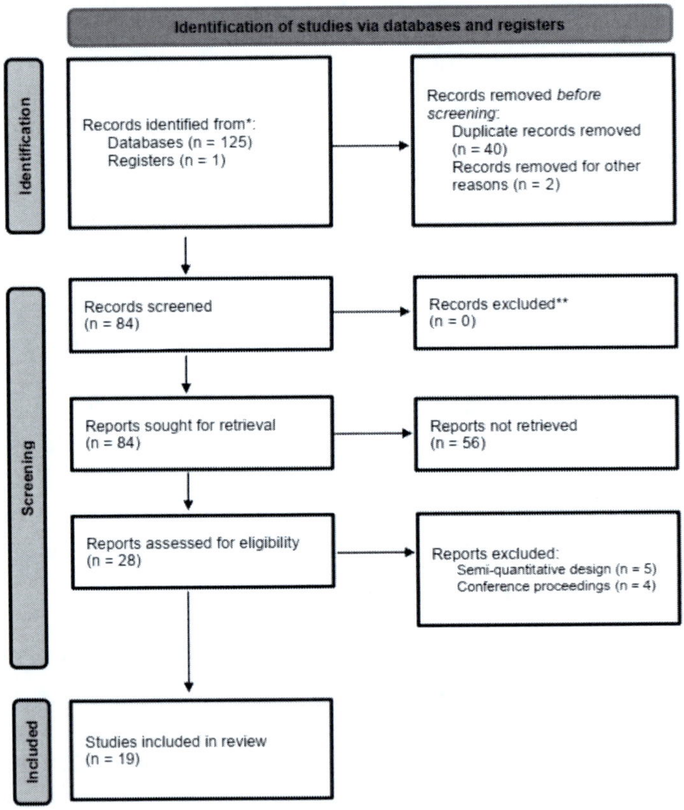

Figure 1. Flow diagram of the study.

Information Sources and Search Strategy

The two authors of this review searched the PubMed, EMBASE, and Cochrane Central Register of Controlled Trials databases. Different search strategies were used to optimize the number of relevant outcomes, including keywords such as "CTPA," "dual energy CT," and "pulmonary embolism." No date or language restrictions were established. We planned to include studies with a publication date later than January 1st, 2012, and the search was updated to April 4, 2022.

All titles and abstracts of interest were screened and those which did not meet the eligibility criteria were excluded. Subsequently, the screened studies were fully read to assess whether they met all eligibility criteria. Figure 1 shows the flow diagram of the study.

Selection of Studies, Data Extraction and Management

The two review authors independently screened the papers identified by the literature search. The two authors of the work independently extracted data from the selected articles and reviewed them together to resolve discrepancies.

Results

Fundamentals of SECT and DECT

SECT, with a single energy polychromatic X-ray beam, provides information on the location of materials and distinguishes them according to their radiological density, measured in Hounsfield Units (HUs). These HUs depend on the linear attenuation coefficient of the voxel, which in turn depends on both the mass attenuation coefficient of the material and the density of the material, so that they provide quantitative information about the density of the material compared to that of water (i.e., 0 HUs). However, it fails to differentiate between two materials that share the same HUs, even I they are materials with very different composition and physical characteristics [17].

The first single-energy scanners were sequential axial acquisition scanners (i.e., CAT scans), which were later replaced by helical acquisition scanners, allowing continuous acquisition during rotation of the X-ray tube and simultaneous movement of the table with the patient, resulting in a shorter scan duration and volumetric imaging [17].

Classically, helical CT scans have been divided into two main types according to the number and arrangement of detectors: single detector helical CT (SDCT) and multi-detector helical CT (MDCT) [18]. The former has a single row of X-ray detectors to record the information as the gantry rotates around the patient, performing a single and continuous spiral acquisition, in which the slice thickness is determined by the degree of collimation of the X-ray beam. MDCT, on the other hand, has multiple rows of detectors parallel to each other (16, 64, 128, and even 320) that record data independently as the gantry rotates and moves forward, obtaining a greater volume of information with less displacement than SDCT.

Currently, helical MDCT or multislice CT has replaced SDCT, since it is faster, requires less acquisition time, and allows images with different slice thicknesses to be reconstructed. In addition, the acquisition of volumetric data and the performance of such thin slices, which can be submillimetric, originates isotropic images that can be studied in the three axes of space with multiplanar and 3D reconstructions without losing spatial resolution [15].

Moreover, the basic differential aspect of DECT and its novel contribution with respect to previous CT modalities consists in the acquisition of the image using two different energy levels of the X-ray beam, measured in kilovoltage peak (kVp).

Tissues show different radiation absorption patterns when subjected to different energy levels, so that two very similar tissues with a similar CT attenuation pattern, such as blood and iodinated contrast, can be differentiated if subjected to two different types of energy, overcoming a major limitation of SECT. Likewise, DECT can be used to improve the signal-to-noise ratio, helping to detect and characterize lesions, reducing noise and image artifacts [19].

Different energy levels have different effects on the image obtained, so that an X-ray beam at lower kVp results in higher tissue absorption and higher iodine density and contrast, but results in a noisier image (lower contrast-to-noise ratio and signal-to-noise ratio). Therefore, the objective of the post-processing techniques will be to combine the greater attenuation of the iodine contrast thanks to a low kVp beam (70-100 kv) with an image that has less noise due to the high kVp beam (140-150 kv) using mainly what is known as Linear Blending (LB) [20]. Other techniques such as material decomposition analysis allow the creation of Iodine Maps (IM), Virtual Monoenergetic Imaging (VMI), Noise-Optimized Virtual Monochromatic Imaging (VMI+), and Virtual Non Contrast (VNC) [21, 22].

However, although the physical basis of DECT is the same, the image acquisition strategies have changed over time and vary according to the different manufacturers. Therefore, there are a wide variety of DECT scanners: those that perform two consecutive scans changing the kVp of the

X-ray beam between one and the other; those that perform a single with a single energy source with fast changes in the kVp of the X-ray beam, using a single polychromatic X-ray source but with specialized multilayer detectors where some rows record low energy information and others record high energy information, arranged as a "sandwich"; and, finally, those that have a double source and double system of detectors [19, 23].

Study Protocol for the Diagnosis of PE and Post-Processing Techniques

The rationale and study protocol for the diagnosis of PE is similar in both SECT and DECT, since they try to demonstrate the intraluminal occupation of the pulmonary arteries by thrombotic material. For this purpose, iodinated intravenous contrast is first administered through a peripheral or central venous line, with a contrast volume of 1 ml/kg body weight and a flow rate of 3 to 4 ml/s. Then, a chest CT is performed, synchronizing the acquisition with the arrival of the contrast bolus to the pulmonary arteries by means of "bolus timing" (injection of contrast approximately 20 seconds before starting the study) or "bolus tracking" (placing a ROI inside the main pulmonary artery trunk that detects the increase in HU due to iodine). Thus, any visible filling defect within a pulmonary artery is usually thrombotic material and diagnostic of PE, although we must not forget that intraluminal masses can also be seen in the case of pulmonary artery sarcoma and tumor embolism [24].

If the patient is young and healthy, the CTPA will be performed while the patient out-breaths, or with free breathing or soft apnea, rather than in forced inspiration to avoid the artifact caused by an excessive increase in intrathoracic pressure [13, 25]. By asking the patient to breathe in prior to the CT scan, as we would do in a conventional chest exploration, we run the risk of a sudden increase in intrathoracic pressure while the bolus of contrast travels through the pulmonary arteries, causing the column of contrast that remains behind not to advance towards the thorax and the one that circulated through the thorax to advance rapidly towards the systemic circuit. As a result we will see intravenous contrast in the systemic circuit and a remnant of the same in the venous route of administration, while the pulmonary arterial tree, object of study, will be slightly opacified.

Subsequently, whether we use SECT or DECT, we can use classical post-processing techniques such as multiplanar and 3D reconstructions, maximum intensity projections (MIPs), and minimum intensity projections (minIPs), as well as specific reconstruction algorithms for the study of the pulmonary parenchyma [17]. However, DECT stands out in the diagnosis of PE due to the possibility of using new postprocessing techniques, which we will proceed to explain.

LB is the most widely used non-material-specific postprocessing method in DECT, consisting of an algorithm that combines the information and advantages offered respectively by a low and high energy level, trying to offer an image with the best signal/noise ratio [21].

On the other hand, there are the two-material and three-material decomposition algorithms. In the case of the "two-material decomposition," it would be calculated what relative amount of iodine versus the acute molecule contributes to the X-ray absorption and attenuation of the image obtained, creating "iodine, no water" and "water, no iodine" maps. Tissues that do not correspond to iodine or water are also decomposed into these two materials, causing their total attenuation to be split between these two groups, in the case of calcium its attenuation is equally divided. In the three-material decomposition, maps would be created this time for calcium as well as for water and iodine. Iodine-based maps of three-material decay are especially useful in the demonstration of PE by creating perfusion maps [23]. Pulmonary perfusion maps depict the distribution of iodine throughout the pulmonary arterial tree, simulating the performance of a perfusion scan, allowing assessment of distal perfusion defects due to PE and increasing sensitivity in the detection of small peripheral pulmonary thrombi [21, 26].

VMI is a post-processing technique that seeks to reconstruct the image of both X-ray beams by determining a hypothetical single energy level, simulating a real SECT. This chosen energy level is called kiloelectronvolt (keV), and the image obtained will be the result of synthesizing the information of both energy levels. At a high keV level, it has been shown that beam hardening artifacts produced by high density material such as metal, contrast enhancement or vascular calcifications decrease. On the contrary, a low keV level allows the interpretation of a study under low contrast level conditions, as it maximizes contrast attenuation, being especially useful in vascular studies such as CTPA and in patients with impaired renal function, allowing to use a smaller amount of contrast and increasing sensitivity in the detection of small thrombi even with poor vascular opacification. The reconstructions at a higher or lower keV must therefore serve the purpose of the study and the patient's characteristics, although fortunately they are reconstructions that can be performed retrospectively [22].

Following VMI, VMI+ arises, which aims to overcome the limitations of VMI by seeking an image with low noise and high iodine contrast, combining the advantages of high and low keV. VMI+ reconstructions have proven to be of high utility in oncology patients undergoing CT with intravenous contrast in portal phase only, in that they achieve image quality in pulmonary vessels capable of ruling out incidental PE. They even achieve an image quality comparable to angiography dedicated to the study of pulmonary arteries [22].

And finally, CNV consists of digital and selective subtraction of the iodine detected in the image, making it possible to obtain images without and with iodinated contrast without the need to acquire the images twice [21].

Diagnostic Findings in PE and Other Findings

CTPA allows to determine the presence or absence of filling defects in the pulmonary arterial tree suggestive of PE, but it will also provide valuable information about it, the involvement of the pulmonary parenchyma and cardiovascular system, and any other concomitant normal or pathological findings.

PTE can be classified according to its chronology as acute, chronic or mixed, since each shows a different radiological appearance. When the thrombus completely occludes an arterial vessel, it shows normal or increased caliber if it is acute, while it decreases in size with a tendency to atrophy if it is chronic. If the thrombus causes a partial obstruction and is acute, it will appear as a central defect in the lumen, being characteristic the "railway track sign" (longitudinal axis) and the "mint pole sign" (axial axis), and also the defect forms acute angles with the vessel wall. If, on the contrary, it causes partial obstruction and is chronic, it will appear as an eccentric defect, adhered to the wall, looking parallel to the wall in the longitudinal axis, forming obtuse angles with the vessel wall [27].

There are also some indirect radiological signs that can guide us to a greater or lesser extent to the suspicion of acute or chronic PE. Acute PE should be suspected when an increase in the size of the pulmonary hila, ground-glass opacities (in probable relation to alveolar hemorrhage foci or surrounding edema), atelectasis, as well as pulmonary infarction (peripheral alveolar condensation focus, of triangular morphology, with a pleural base and non-enhancing) are observed. On the other hand, chronic PE should be suspected when signs of recanalization are observed (e.g., bands, networks, membranes, areas of stenosis, areas of architectural distortion or calcifications), mosaic pattern (i.e., areas of hypo- and hyperperfusion), increased caliber of bronchial arteries and collaterals originating in the intercostal arteries, as well as indirect signs suggestive of pulmonary hypertension, e.g., an increase in the axial diameter of the pulmonary artery trunk (>28 mm) [27].

CTPA can also allow to classify PE according to its location and extension, as central if it affects main and lobar branches, or peripheral if it only affects segmental and subsegmental branches. Moreover, early signs of complications due to PE such as right heart strain [5], manifested by an increase in the size of the right chambers (RV/LV ratio < 0.9 and RA > 3.5cm), rectification or inversion of the interventricular septum, reflux of iodinated contrast to the inferior vena cava and hepatic veins, and abnormal dilatation of the azygos vein, in addition to other complications such as pulmonary infarction, pericardial or pleural effusion, and atelectasis. But it is also capable of showing other thoracic pathologic findings such as chronic obstructive pulmonary disease, signs suggestive of interstitial diffuse pulmonary disease, tracheobronchial alterations, enlarged lymph nodes, pulmonary nodules or masses.

Therefore, in young and presumably healthy patients in whom we are not going to perform forced inspiration to avoid the defect of focal opacification of the pulmonary arterial tree, it may be necessary to schedule a previous acquisition without intravenous contrast and in inspiration that allows an adequate assessment of concomitant pulmonary pathology [13].

However, CTPA is not free of risks and limitations. These include the radiation dose (usually 3-10 mSv), a limiting factor in pregnant and young women due to greater radiosensitivity, and the need to administer iodinated contrast, contraindicated in patients with impaired kidney function and limited in pregnant women, people allergic to iodine, or hyperthyroid patients [1].

Comparison between SDCT and DECT

There are two recent meta-analyses that evaluate the performance of DECT in the diagnosis of PE; Abdellatif et al. (2021) reported sensitivity and specificity values of 88.9% and 94.6%, respectively, while Monti et al. (2021) reported both values at approximately 90% [28, 29]. Such sensitivity and specificity values of DECT are not far from those observed in SECT (83% and 96%, respectively) in the PIOPED II study [14]. All the studies reported use different types of DECT technology. In the meta-analysis conducted by Abdellatif et al. [29], 7 studies [30-36] were included (Table 1), most of them of small sample size. In the meta-analysis by Monti CB et al. (28), 17 studies [31, 33-48] were included (Table 2). However, this meta-analysis only evaluated the results of DECT in the diagnosis of acute PE with lobar and segmental involvement since there were insufficient data to compare both techniques in the case of chronic or subsegmental PE. Some of the studies only analyzed the performance of LB alone [35, 38, 43-45, 47], in others LB together with IM [31, 33-35, 37-43, 46, 47] and others the joint performance of the three techniques (i.e., LB, IM and VM) [43, 48].

Table 1. Studies analyzing the performance of dual-energy computed tomography in the diagnosis of pulmonary embolism in the meta-analysis Abdellatif et al. (2021). P, prospective. R, retrospective

Number	Name of the study	Year	Study design	N
1	Thieme et al. 2008	2008	P	13
2	Fink et al. 2008	2008	P	24
3	Zhang et al. 2009	2009	R	31
4	Lee et al. 2011	2011	R	37
5	Geyer et al. 2012	2012	R	14
6	Miura et al. 2015	2015	R	13
7	Zhang et al. 2018	2018	P	50

Adapted from Abdellatif W, Ebada MA, Alkanj S, Negida A, Murray N, Khosa F, et al. Diagnostic Accuracy of Dual-Energy CT in Detection of Acute Pulmonary Embolism: A Systematic Review and Meta-Analysis. Canadian Association of Radiologists Journal. 2021 May 1;72(2):285–92.

Within this larger meta-analysis, the studies presented by Okada et al. (2018), Thieme et al. (2014), Geyer et al. (2012), Bauer et al. (2011), Thieme et al. (2008) and Weiss et al. (2017) are the ones that move further away from the sensitivity provided by SECT, some of them for having very large confidence intervals in probable relation to a low sample size [33, 34, 39, 42, 45, 46], in no case exceeding 0.83 sensitivity. On the other hand, those presenting a lower specificity with respect to SECT are those presented by Thieme et al. (2014), Sueyoshi et al. (2011), and Thieme et al. (2008), the latter having a large confidence interval, and none of them exceeding 0.87 specificity.

Table 2. Studies analyzing the performance of dual-energy computed tomography in the diagnosis of pulmonary embolism in the meta-analysis Monti et al. (2021). P, prospective. R, retrospective

Number	Name of the study	Year	Country	Study design	N
1	Kroger et al. 2019	2019	Germany	R	60
2	Grob et al. 2019	2019	The Netherlands	P	75
3	Masy et al. 2019	2019	France	R	80
4	Okada et al. 2018	2018	Japan	R	168
5	Leithner et al. 2017	2017	USA	R	68
6	Weiss et al. 2017	2017	Germany	R	52
7	Li et al. 2017	2017	China	P	33
8	Cai et al. 2015	2015	China	P	76
9	Okada et al. 2015	2015	Japan	R	83
10	Thieme et al. 2014	2014	Germany	R	232
11	Geyer et al. 2012	2012	Germany	R	14
12	Sueyoshi et al. 2011	2011	Japan	P	113
13	Bauer et al. 2011	2011	Germany	R	9
14	Lee et al. 2011	2011	Republic of Korea	R	37
15	Zhang et al. 2009	2009	China	P	31
16	Fink et al. 2008	2008	Germany	P	24
17	Thieme et al. 2008	2008	Germany	P	13

Adapted from Monti CB, Zanardo M, Cozzi A, Schiaffino S, Spagnolo P, Secchi F, et al. Dual-energy CT performance in acute pulmonary embolism: a meta-analysis. European Radiology. 2021 Aug 1;31(8):6248–58.

The rest of the studies, and in general when all the studies are analyzed together, yield very similar results to those found in SECT. Accordingly, despite the novel DECT postprocessing techniques, there do not seem to be major differences in the performance of both types of CTPA in the diagnosis of acute lobar or segmental PE. Of note, DECT studies seem to generate an increase in the time and complexity of the reconstructions and of the correct reading of the study, and may result in an increased workload for the radiologist [28]. However, not enough data are available on the comparison between the performance of DECT and SECT in the diagnosis of chronic and peripheral PE, situations in which DECT could offer certain advantages. Future studies are therefore warranted on this topic.

Conclusion

Single- and dual-energy multidetector computed tomography show similar sensitivity and specificity in the diagnosis of acute lobar and segmental PE.

However, insufficient data concerning the diagnosis of chronic and subsegmental PE are yet available.

The advantage of DECT is that it allows the administration of a smaller volume of iodinated contrast and involves a lower dose of ionizing radiation, although more studies are needed to investigate the cost-effectiveness of DECT versus SECT.

References

[1] Konstantinides, S. V., Meyer, G., Becattini, C., Bueno, H., Geersing, G. J., Harjola, V. P., Huisman, M. V., Humbert, M., Jennings, C. S., Jiménez, D., Kucher, N., Lang, I. M., Lankeit, M., Lorusso, R., Mazzolai, L., Meneveau, N., Ní Áinle, F., Prandoni, P., Pruszczyk, P., Righini, M., ... ESC Scientific Document Group (2020). 2019 ESC Guidelines for the diagnosis and management of acute pulmonary embolism developed in collaboration with the European Respiratory Society (ERS). *European Heart Journal*, *41*(4), 543–603. https://doi.org/10.1093/ eurheartj/ehz405.

[2] Duffett, L., Castellucci, L. A., & Forgie, M. A. (2020). Pulmonary embolism: update on management and controversies. *BMJ (Clinical Research Ed.)*, *370*, m2177. https://doi.org/10.1136/bmj.m2177.

[3] Thompson, T., & Kabrhel, C. *Overview of Acute Pulmonary Embolism in Adults*. 2022. Available from: https://www.uptodate.com/contents/overview-of-acute-pulmonary-embolism-in-adults/printwww.uptodate.com.

[4] Roy, P. M., Douillet, D., & Penaloza, A. (2021). Contemporary management of acute pulmonary embolism. *Trends in Cardiovascular Medicine*, S1050-1738(21) 00068-2. Advance online publication. https://doi.org/10.1016/j.tcm. 2021.06.002.

[5] Sista, A. K., Kuo, W. T., Schiebler, M., & Madoff, D. C. (2017). Stratification, Imaging, and Management of Acute Massive and Submassive Pulmonary Embolism. *Radiology*, *284*(1), 5–24. https://doi.org/10.1148/radiol.2017151978.

[6] Doherty S. (2017). Pulmonary embolism an update. *Australian Family Physician*, *46*(11), 816–820.

[7] Raja, A. S., Greenberg, J. O., Qaseem, A., Denberg, T. D., Fitterman, N., Schuur, J. D., & Clinical Guidelines Committee of the American College of Physicians (2015). Evaluation of Patients with Suspected Acute Pulmonary Embolism: Best Practice Advice From the Clinical Guidelines Committee of the American College of Physicians. *Annals of Internal Medicine*, *163*(9), 701–711. https://doi.org/10.7326/ M14-1772.

[8] Láinez-Ramos-Bossini, A. J., Moreno-Suárez, S., Pérez-García, M. C., Gálvez-López, R., Sanz, F. G., & Rivera-Izquierdo, M. (2020). Acute pulmonary embolism: appropriateness of emergency department management according to clinical guidelines. Tromboembolismo pulmonar agudo: adecuación del manejo de pacientes según las guías de práctica clínica en el servicio de urgencias. *Radiologia*,

S0033-8338(20)30111-9. Advance online publication. https://doi.org/10.1016/j.rx.2020.06.004.

[9] Láinez-Ramos-Bossini, A. J., Moreno-Suárez, S., Pérez-García, M., Gálvez-López, R., Garrido-Sanz, F., & Rivera-Izquierdo, M. (2020). Use of clinical probability scores and D-dimer in suspected pulmonary embolism. Results from a Spanish retrospective study. *European Journal of Emergency Medicine: Official Journal of the European Society for Emergency Medicine*, *27*(6), 468–469. https://doi.org/10.1097/MEJ.0000000000000722.

[10] Lozano-Polo, L., Puig-Campmany, M., Herrera-Mateo, S., Mateo-Roca, M., Santos-Rodríguez, J. A., & Benito-Vales, S. (2018). Diagnosis of pulmonary embolism in the elderly: adherence to guidelines and age-adjusted D-dimer concentration values. *Emergencias: Revista de la Sociedad Espanola de Medicina de Emergencias*, *30*(5), 321–327.

[11] Molaee, S., Ghanaati, H., Safavi, E., Foroumandi, M., & Peiman, S. (2015). Computed Tomography Pulmonary Angiography for Evaluation of Patients With Suspected Pulmonary Embolism: Use or Overuse. *Iranian Journal of Radiology: A Quarterly Journal Published by the Iranian Radiological Society*, *12*(3), e22383. https://doi.org/10.5812/iranjradiol.12(2)2015.22383.

[12] Howard L. (2019). Acute pulmonary embolism. *Clinical Medicine (London, England)*, *19*(3), 243–247. https://doi.org/10.7861/clinmedicine.19-3-247.

[13] Tilve-Gómez, A., Rodríguez-Fernández, P., Trillo-Fandiño, L., & Plasencia-Martínez, J. M. (2017). Imaging techniques used in the diagnostic workup of acute venous thromboembolic disease. *Radiologia*, *59*(4), 329–342. https://doi.org/10.1016/j.rx.2016.10.003.

[14] Stein, P. D., Fowler, S. E., Goodman, L. R., Gottschalk, A., Hales, C. A., Hull, R. D., Leeper, K. V., Jr, Popovich, J., Jr, Quinn, D. A., Sos, T. A., Sostman, H. D., Tapson, V. F., Wakefield, T. W., Weg, J. G., Woodard, P. K., & PIOPED II Investigators (2006). Multidetector computed tomography for acute pulmonary embolism. *The New England Journal of Medicine*, *354*(22), 2317–2327. https://doi.org/10.1056/NEJMoa052367.

[15] Láinez Ramos-Bossini, A. J., Salmerón-Ruiz, Á., Martínez Barbero, J. P., Martín Molina, J. P., Martín Rodríguez, J. L., López Milena, G., & Ruiz Santiago, F. Cross-sectional correlate for integrative imaging (anatomical radiology). In: *Gholamrezanezhad A, Assadi M, Jadvar H. Multidisciplinary Diagnostic Imaging: Radiology-Nuclear Medicine Correlative Imaging*. Wiley-Blackwell. ISBN-10: 1119603617.

[16] Page, M. J., McKenzie, J. E., Bossuyt, P. M., Boutron, I., Hoffmann, T. C., Mulrow, C. D., Shamseer, L., Tetzlaff, J. M., Akl, E. A., Brennan, S. E., Chou, R., Glanville, J., Grimshaw, J. M., Hróbjartsson, A., Lalu, M. M., Li, T., Loder, E. W., Mayo-Wilson, E., McDonald, S., McGuinness, L. A., … Moher, D. (2021). The PRISMA 2020 statement: an updated guideline for reporting systematic reviews. *BMJ (Clinical Research ed.)*, *372*, n71. https://doi.org/10.1136/bmj.n71.

[17] Little B. P. (2015). Approach to chest computed tomography. *Clinics in Chest Medicine*, 36(2), 127–vii. https://doi.org/10.1016/j.ccm.2015.02.001.

[18] Webb, R., Brant, W., & Major, N. *Fundamentals of Body CT*, 5th Ed. New York, New York: Elsevier Inc.; 2019.

[19] Siegel, M. J., Kaza, R. K., Bolus, D. N., Boll, D. T., Rofsky, N. M., De Cecco, C. N., Foley, W. D., Morgan, D. E., Schoepf, U. J., Sahani, D. V., Shuman, W. P., Vrtiska, T. J., Yeh, B. M., & Berland, L. L. (2016). White Paper of the Society of Computed Body Tomography and Magnetic Resonance on Dual-Energy CT, Part 1: Technology and Terminology. *Journal of Computer Assisted Tomography*, 40(6), 841–845. https://doi.org/10.1097/RCT.0000000000000531.

[20] Johnson T. R. (2012). Dual-energy CT: general principles. *AJR. American Journal of Roentgenology*, *199*(5 Suppl), S3–S8. https://doi.org/10.2214/AJR.12.9116.

[21] Martin, S. S., van Assen, M., Griffith, L. P., de Cecco, C. N., Varga-Szemes, A., Bauer, M. J., Wichmann, J. L., Vogl, T. L. & Schoepf, U. J. (2018). Dual-Energy CT Pulmonary Angiography: Quantification of Disease Burden and Impact on Management. *Current Radiology Reports*. Springer New York LLC. https://inis.iaea.org/search/search.aspx?orig_q=RN:51038395.

[22] D'Angelo, T., Cicero, G., Mazziotti, S., Ascenti, G., Albrecht, M. H., Martin, S. S., Othman, A. E., Vogl, T. J., & Wichmann, J. L. (2019). Dual energy computed tomography virtual monoenergetic imaging: technique and clinical applications. *The British Journal of Radiology*, *92*(1098), 20180546. https://doi.org/10.1259/ bjr.20180546.

[23] McCollough CH, Leng S, Yu L, Fletcher JG. Dual- and multi-energy CT: Principles, technical approaches, and clinical applications. *Radiology*. 2015 Sep 1;276(3):637–53.

[24] Webb R, Brant W, Major N. Mediastinum: vascular abnormalities. In: *Fundamentals of Body CT*. 3rd Ed. New York: Elsevier Inc.; 2007. p. 45–7.

[25] Raczeck, P., Minko, P., Graeber, S., Fries, P., Seidel, R., Buecker, A., & Stroeder, J. (2016). Influence of Respiratory Position on Contrast Attenuation in Pulmonary CT Angiography: A Prospective Randomized Clinical Trial. *AJR. American Journal of Roentgenology*, *206*(3), 481–486. https://doi.org/10.2214/AJR.15.15176.

[26] Okada, M., Kunihiro, Y., Nakashima, Y., Nomura, T., Kudomi, S., Yonezawa, T., Suga, K., & Matsunaga, N. (2015). Added value of lung perfused blood volume images using dual-energy CT for assessment of acute pulmonary embolism. *European Journal of Radiology*, *84*(1), 172–177. https://doi.org/10.1016/j.ejrad.2014.09.009.

[27] Wittram, C., Maher, M. M., Yoo, A. J., Kalra, M. K., Shepard, J. A., & McLoud, T. C. (2004). CT angiography of pulmonary embolism: diagnostic criteria and causes of misdiagnosis. *Radiographics: A Review Publication of the Radiological Society of North America, Inc*, *24*(5), 1219–1238. https://doi.org/10.1148/rg. 245045008.

[28] Monti, C. B., Zanardo, M., Cozzi, A., Schiaffino, S., Spagnolo, P., Secchi, F., De Cecco, C. N., & Sardanelli, F. (2021). Dual-energy CT performance in acute pulmonary embolism: a meta-analysis. *European Radiology*, *31*(8), 6248–6258. https://doi.org/10.1007/s00330-020-07633-8.

[29] Abdellatif, W., Ebada, M. A., Alkanj, S., Negida, A., Murray, N., Khosa, F., & Nicolaou, S. (2021). Diagnostic Accuracy of Dual-Energy CT in Detection of Acute Pulmonary Embolism: A Systematic Review and Meta-Analysis. *Canadian*

Association of Radiologists Journal, *72*(2), 285–292. https://doi.org/10.1177/0846537120902062.

[30] Miura, S., Ohno, Y., Kimura, H., & Kichikawa, K. (2015). Quantitative lung perfused blood volume imaging on dual-energy CT: capability for quantitative assessment of disease severity in patients with acute pulmonary thromboembolism. *Acta Radiologica (Stockholm, Sweden: 1987)*, *56*(3), 284–293. https://doi.org/10.1177/0284185114524953.

[31] Zhang, L. J., Yang, G. F., Zhao, Y. E., Zhou, C. S., & Lu, G. M. (2009). Detection of pulmonary embolism using dual-energy computed tomography and correlation with cardiovascular measurements: a preliminary study. *Acta radiologica (Stockholm, Sweden: 1987)*, *50*(8), 892–901. https://doi.org/10.1080/02841850903095393.

[32] Zhang, J., Cai, J., Liu, S., & Zhang, X. (2018). Value of Dual-energy Lung Perfusion Imaging Using a Dual-source CT System for the Pulmonary Embolism. *Open Life Sciences*, *13*, 107–111. https://doi.org/10.1515/biol-2018-0015.

[33] Thieme, S. F., Becker, C. R., Hacker, M., Nikolaou, K., Reiser, M. F., & Johnson, T. R. (2008). Dual energy CT for the assessment of lung perfusion--correlation to scintigraphy. *European Journal of Radiology*, *68*(3), 369–374. https://doi.org/10.1016/j.ejrad.2008.07.031.

[34] Geyer, L. L., Scherr, M., Körner, M., Wirth, S., Deak, P., Reiser, M. F., & Linsenmaier, U. (2012). Imaging of acute pulmonary embolism using a dual energy CT system with rapid kVp switching: initial results. *European Journal of Radiology*, *81*(12), 3711–3718. https://doi.org/10.1016/j.ejrad.2011.02.043.

[35] Lee, C. W., Seo, J. B., Song, J. W., Kim, M. Y., Lee, H. Y., Park, Y. S., Chae, E. J., Jang, Y. M., Kim, N., & Krauss, B. (2011). Evaluation of computer-aided detection and dual energy software in detection of peripheral pulmonary embolism on dual-energy pulmonary CT angiography. *European radiology*, *21*(1), 54–62. https://doi.org/10.1007/s00330-010-1903-7.

[36] Fink, C., Johnson, T. R., Michaely, H. J., Morhard, D., Becker, C., Reiser, M., & Nikolaou, K. (2008). Dual-energy CT angiography of the lung in patients with suspected pulmonary embolism: initial results. *RoFo: Fortschritte auf dem Gebiete der Rontgenstrahlen und der Nuklearmedizin*, *180*(10), 879–883. https://doi.org/10.1055/s-2008-1027724.

[37] Kröger, J. R., Gerhardt, F., Dumitrescu, D., Rosenkranz, S., Schmidt, M., Maintz, D., & Bunck, A. C. (2019). Diagnosis of pulmonary hypertension using spectral-detector CT. *International Journal of Cardiology*, *285*, 80–85. https://doi.org/10.1016/j.ijcard.2019.03.018.

[38] Grob, D., Smit, E., Prince, J., Kist, J., Stöger, L., Geurts, B., Snoeren, M. M., van Dijk, R., Oostveen, L. J., Prokop, M., Schaefer-Prokop, C. M., Sechopoulos, I., & Brink, M. (2019). Iodine Maps from Subtraction CT or Dual-Energy CT to Detect Pulmonary Emboli with CT Angiography: A Multiple-Observer Study. *Radiology*, *292*(1), 197–205. https://doi.org/10.1148/radiol.2019182666.

[39] Bauer, R. W., Kerl, J. M., Weber, E., Weisser, P., Korkusuz, H., Lehnert, T., Jacobi, V., & Vogl, T. J. (2011). Lung perfusion analysis with dual energy CT in patients with suspected pulmonary embolism--influence of window settings on the diagnosis

of underlying pathologies of perfusion defects. *European Journal of Radiology, 80*(3), e476–e482. https://doi.org/10.1016/j.ejrad.2010.09.009.

[40] Sueyoshi, E., Tsutsui, S., Hayashida, T., Ashizawa, K., Sakamoto, I., & Uetani, M. (2011). Quantification of lung perfusion blood volume (lung PBV) by dual-energy CT in patients with and without pulmonary embolism: preliminary results. *European Journal of Radiology, 80*(3), e505–e509. https://doi.org/10.1016/j.ejrad.2010.10.011.

[41] Masy, M., Giordano, J., Petyt, G., Hossein-Foucher, C., Duhamel, A., Kyheng, M., De Groote, P., Fertin, M., Lamblin, N., Bervar, J. F., Remy, J., & Remy-Jardin, M. (2018). Dual-energy CT (DECT) lung perfusion in pulmonary hypertension: concordance rate with V/Q scintigraphy in diagnosing chronic thromboembolic pulmonary hypertension (CTEPH). *European Radiology, 28*(12), 5100–5110. https://doi.org/10.1007/s00330-018-5467-2.

[42] Okada, M., Nomura, T., Nakashima, Y., Kunihiro, Y., & Kido, S. (2018). Histogram-pattern analysis of the lung perfused blood volume for assessment of pulmonary thromboembolism. *Diagnostic and Interventional Radiology (Ankara, Turkey), 24*(3), 139–145. https://doi.org/10.5152/dir.2018.17311.

[43] Leithner, D., Wichmann, J. L., Vogl, T. J., Trommer, J., Martin, S. S., Scholtz, J. E., Bodelle, B., De Cecco, C. N., Duguay, T., Nance, J. W., Jr, Schoepf, U. J., & Albrecht, M. H. (2017). Virtual Monoenergetic Imaging and Iodine Perfusion Maps Improve Diagnostic Accuracy of Dual-Energy Computed Tomography Pulmonary Angiography With Suboptimal Contrast Attenuation. *Investigative Radiology, 52*(11), 659–665. https://doi.org/10.1097/RLI.0000000000000387.

[44] Li, X., Chen, G. Z., Zhao, Y. E., Schoepf, U. J., Albrecht, M. H., Bickford, M. W., Gu, H. F., Zhang, L. J., & Lu, G. M. (2017). Radiation Optimized Dual-source Dual-energy Computed Tomography Pulmonary Angiography: Intra-individual and Inter-individual Comparison. *Academic Radiology, 24*(1), 13–21. https://doi.org/10.1016/j.acra.2016.09.009.

[45] Weiss, J., Notohamiprodjo, M., Bongers, M., Schabel, C., Mangold, S., Nikolaou, K., Bamberg, F., & Othman, A. E. (2017). Effect of Noise-Optimized Monoenergetic Postprocessing on Diagnostic Accuracy for Detecting Incidental Pulmonary Embolism in Portal-Venous Phase Dual-Energy Computed Tomography. *Investigative Radiology, 52*(3), 142–147. https://doi.org/10.1097/RLI.0000000000000319.

[46] Thieme, S. F., Meinel, F. G., Graef, A., Helck, A. D., Reiser, M. F., & Johnson, T. R. (2014). Dual-energy CT pulmonary angiography in patients with suspected pulmonary embolism: value for the detection and quantification of pulmonary venous congestion. *The British Journal of Radiology, 87*(1039), 20140079. https://doi.org/10.1259/bjr.20140079.

[47] Okada, M., Kunihiro, Y., Nakashima, Y., Nomura, T., Kudomi, S., Yonezawa, T., Suga, K., & Matsunaga, N. (2015). Added value of lung perfused blood volume images using dual-energy CT for assessment of acute pulmonary embolism. *European Journal of Radiology, 84*(1), 172–177. https://doi.org/10.1016/j.ejrad.2014.09.009.

[48] Cai, X. R., Feng, Y. Z., Qiu, L., Xian, Z. H., Yang, W. C., Mo, X. K., & Wang, X. B. (2015). Iodine Distribution Map in Dual-Energy Computed Tomography Pulmonary Artery Imaging with Rapid kVp Switching for the Diagnostic Analysis and Quantitative Evaluation of Acute Pulmonary Embolism. *Academic Radiology*, *22*(6), 743–751. https://doi.org/10.1016/j.acra.2015.01.012.

Chapter 3

Diagnosis of Pulmonary Embolism in Clinical Practice. Status Quo Prior to the COVID-19 Pandemic in Southern Spain

Antonio Jesús Láinez Ramos-Bossini, MD[1,2,3]
[1]Department of Radiology,
Hospital Universitario Virgen de las Nieves,
Granada, Spain
[2]Biosanitary Research Institute, Granada, Spain
[3]Department of Psychiatry, School of Medicine,
University of Granada, Granada, Spain

Abstract

The aim of this study was to evaluate the use of clinical probability scores and several factors related to the diagnosis of pulmonary embolism (PE) in patients that underwent computed tomography chest angiography (CTCA) for suspected PE at the emergency department (ED) in our institution. Retrospective observational study addressing the CTCAs ordered for suspected PE in our ED during 2018. Epidemiological, clinical and analytical factors, as well as the use of clinical probability scores (CPS), were analyzed. Two-level Wells score (WS), revised Geneva score (GS) and their simplified versions (sWS and sGS, respectively) were retrospectively calculated, and guideline adherence was analyzed accordingly.

In total, 534 patients (52.8% women, median age: 73 years) were included. The frequency of PE was 23.0%. The WS had been explicitly applied in 15.2% of all cases. Significant differences were found between retrospective CPSs (PE likely: WS (12.9%); sWS (26.4%); GS (45.5%); sGS (43.4%); $p < 0.001$). D-dimer tests were ordered in 88.2% of all cases (97.6% and 93.4% were positive, according to the standard and age-adjusted upper limits, respectively). Lack of adherence to guidelines

In: Understanding and Treating Acute Pulmonary Embolism
Editor: James K. Edwards
ISBN: 979-8-88697-149-1

varied between CPSs (WS: 15.6%; sWS: 24.0%; GS: 40.3%; sGS: 39.0%).

In conclusion, a poor explicit use of the WS was observed in our study. Our results suggest that the yield of clinical gestalt assessment might be similar to that of CPSs. However, specific studies are further required to verify our findings.

Keywords: pulmonary embolism, computed tomography angiography, guideline adherence, clinical probability scales, Wells criteria, Geneva scale, D-dimer

Introduction

Acute pulmonary embolism (PE) is a relatively common medical emergency with considerable morbidity and mortality, only surpassed by myocardial ischemia and stroke (Alfonso Figueredo et al., 2016; Sandoval B. & Florenzano V., 2015). There are no significant differences regarding sex, and PE prevalence increases with age (Alfonso Figueredo et al., 2016; Guijarro Merino et al., 2008; Lozano-Polo et al., 2018). The clinical presentation of PE encompasses a wide spectrum of signs and symptoms, and routine exams at the Emergency Department (ED), e.g., EKG, X-rays, blood analysis, have low specificity for its detection. Therefore, specific diagnostic exams are required. Computed tomography chest angiography (CTCA) is the technique of choice to diagnose PE and also allows to rule out alternative diagnoses (Konstantinides et al., 2019; Moores et al., 2016; Sandoval B. & Florenzano V., 2015). However, this imaging technique involves significant costs, radiation exposure, and possible contrast-induced nephropathy. Therefore, risks and benefits must be thoroughly weighed before ordering a CTCA to rule out PE (Sanjuán et al., 2014; Van Es, 2017).

Despite the progress made in PE diagnosis, its prognosis has not improved in a parallel manner, and only a slight decrease in mortality has been reported in recent years (Jiménez et al., 2016; Maestre Peiró et al., 2017). To help with risk assessment of PE and appropriate decision making, several clinical probability scales (CPSs) have been developed and validated, including the Wells Score (WS) and the revised Geneva Score (GS) (Raja et al., 2015; Tritschler et al., 2018). Simplified versions of these CPSs have also been developed and validated, and they have proved to have a similar yield compared to the respective extended scores (Douma et al., 2011; Van Es, 2017). Currently, the combination of any validated CPS and serum levels of

D-dimer (DD) is recommended by international guidelines to order a CTCA. However, the low explicit use of CPSs in the ED has been reported across many countries (Lozano-Polo et al., 2018; Molaee et al., 2015; Sanjuán et al., 2014).

Poor adherence to the use of CPSs in routine medical practice has been linked to negative consequences, including unnecessary medical exams, increased healthcare costs, delays in patient attention care, and higher morbidity and mortality rates (Raja et al., 2015). Unfortunately, the application of CPSs in the ED is low, and it has been found to be biased depending on the patients' age (Lozano-Polo et al., 2018). The underlying reasons remain unclear, but differences among studies in terms of sociodemographic variables, PE prevalence, and CTCA yield –especially when comparing European and North American cohorts- might be of importance. In Spain, adherence to clinical guidelines and its impact on the diagnosis of PE have been poorly studied to present. In this work, we aim to analyze the explicit use of WS, adherence to clinical guidelines according to the retrospective estimation of CPSs, and other factors involved in the diagnosis of PE in patients undergoing CTCA for suspected PE at the ED in our hospital.

Methods

This is a retrospective observational study (case series). All cases were selected from the registry of CTCAs performed in the ED of our hospital from January 1st to December 31st, 2018. All CTCAs ordered from the ED were included in the study. Exclusion criteria were age below 18 years old, hemodynamic instability, technical inadequacy of the CTCA, suspicion other than PE, absence of clinical justification in the electronic order, and unavailability of the medical record of the episode. The study was approved by our Institutional Review Board. Figure 1 shows the flow diagram followed during the study.

Recording of the WS -the CPS used in our ED- in the electronic CTCA order or medical record, PE prevalence, and PE subtype were collected. Patient-related variables were also collected, including sociodemographic -age and sex-, vital constants at ED admission (heart rate, blood pressure, arterial oxygen saturation, temperature), cardiovascular risk factors (diabetes mellitus, obesity, hypertension, dyslipidemia, active smoking), main symptoms (dyspnea, cough, syncope, chest pain, hemoptysis, signs of deep venous thrombosis), DD value, final diagnosis, and discharge destination (home, hospital admission, transfer to another hospital or death).

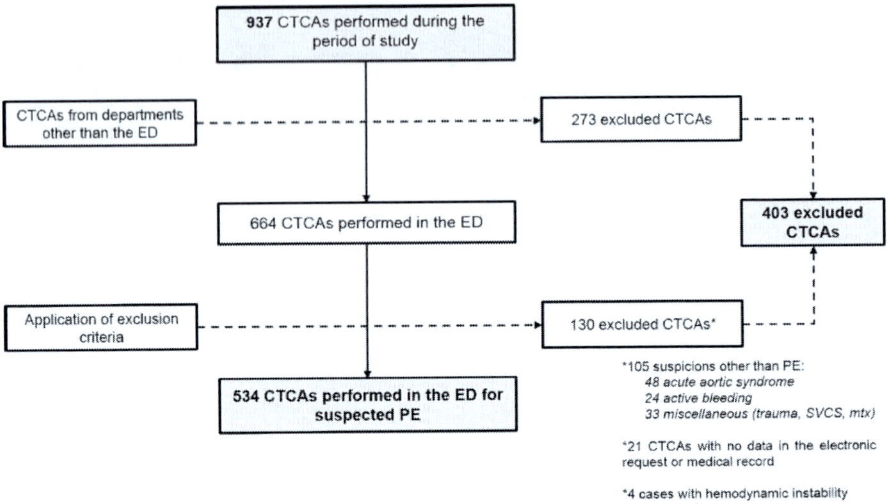

Figure 1. Flow diagram followed in the study. ED: Emergency Department. CTCA: Computed Tomography Chest Angiography. SVCS: Superior Vena Cava Syndrome. Mtx: Metastases.

In our hospital, the DD value is obtained using the ELISA method, which is considered the gold standard (Uresandi et al., 2013), with a standard cut-off value of 500 ng/ml. In patients over 50 years old, age-adjusted DD (aDD) values and its associated intrinsic and extrinsic validity parameters were calculated using the following formula (Marc Righini et al., 2014): age (years) x 10 ng/ml.

Adherence to clinical guidelines was assessed according to internationally validated algorithms (Cronin & Dwamena, 2018; Konstantinides et al., 2019; Uresandi et al., 2013), which are based on risk stratification using any validated CPS and DD value. Two-level risk assessment allows the stratification of PE risk into "PE-likely" or "PE-unlikely". CTCA is indicated if a positive DD value is obtained in the former group, and always in the latter (in which DD should not be ordered). WS, GS and their simplified versions (sWS and sGS, respectively) were retrospectively calculated using data from medical records. Finally, adequate decision-making based on risk stratification was assessed for each CPS.

Table 1. Sociodemographic data of patients, frequency and distribution of pulmonary embolism and D-dimer tests in the sample

Variable	N (%)
Sex	
Male	252 (47.2)
Female	282 (52.8)
Age groups	
≤50	74 (13.9)
51-64	106 (19.9)
65-74	112 (21.0)
75-84	130 (24.3)
85-90	71 (13.3)
≥90	41 (7.7)
Two-level age groups	
<65	186 (34.8)
≥65	348 (65.2)

Variable	Median	Range	Interquartile range	X ± s.d.
Age	73	18-101	24	69.56 ± 17.07

Diagnosis of PE	
CTCA +	123 (23)
CTCA -	411 (77)
Early mortality (<6 months) in patients with PE	19 (15.4)
CPS present in the medical record	81 (15.2)
PE subtype	
Central	68 (12.7)
Peripheral (Segmentary)	47 (8.8)
Peripheral (subsegmentary)	8 (1.5)
Total D-dimer tests in the sample	
Ordered	471 (88.2)
Not ordered	63 (11.8)

CTCA: Computed Tomography Chest Angiography

All cases were collected in an anonymized database. Qualitative variables were expressed in absolute and relative frequencies. Continuous quantitative variables were expressed as mean and standard deviation. Age groups were established according to sociodemographic data (Lozano-Polo et al., 2018). Uni- and bivariate analyses of the collected variables were performed for each age group and according to the presence of PE. Student's t-tests and chi-squared tests were applied after verifying that the conditions for their application were met. Non-parametric tests were applied otherwise. Significance was established at p-values <0.05. IBM SPSS Statistics v. 22.0 for Windows was used for statistical analyses.

Results

Sample Description and Prevalence of Pulmonary Embolism

After applying the exclusion criteria (Figure 1), 534 CTCAs were included in the study (52.8% females). The median age was 73 years (interquartile range: 18-101). PE prevalence was 23.0%. WSs were present in the medical record or in the electronic order in 15.2% of cases. A more detailed analysis of these data is shown in Table 1.

Retrospective Calculation of Clinical Probability Scales and D-Dimer Values

Table 2 shows the retrospective values of all CPSs, as well as the total number of DD tests ordered. In total, 9.8% of cases in which the WS had been explicitly calculated -and thus classified into any risk-category (i.e., PE-likely or PE-unlikely)-, were classified into a different category according to the retrospective WS. Significant differences among all scales were observed depending on the presence of PE.

Of all serum DD tests ordered, 13.2% were not justified according to the risk category group established by the retrospective WS. Among the serum DD tests that were justified, 398 (95.44%) were positive according to the standard cut-off value. After age-adjustment, the number of cases with a negative DD increased to 27 cases. A comparison of the parameters of validity between DD and aDD is shown in Table 3.

Risk Factors, Clinical Presentation, and Final Diagnosis

Table 4 shows the risk factors, comorbidities, symptoms, final diagnosis, and discharge destination for each age group and according to the presence or absence of PE. Notably, almost one-third of all the diagnoses were classified into a miscellaneous category (e.g., pneumothorax, pleural effusion, anxiety, rib fracture, ascites, or sepsis).

Table 2. Retrospective clinical probability scores, PE frequency, and DD tests. Cut-offs for each PE risk group were the same as in Douma et al. [18]

Score	N (%)[a]	PE frequency	P-value (PE vs Non-PE)[b]	D-dimer tests N (%)[b]	CTCA unjustified according to standard D-dimer value	CTCA unjustified according to aDD[c]	Difference between DD and aDD[d]
WS PE-unlikely	465 (87.1)	98 (21.1)	p = .009	409 (88.0)	11 (2.4)	27 (6.6)	16 (4.2)
WS PE-likely	69 (12.9)	25 (36.2)		62 (90.0)	-	-	-
sWS PE-unlikely	393 (73.6)	73 (18.6)	p < .001	352 (89.6)	9 (2.3)	23 (6.5)	14 (4.2)
sWS PE-likely	141 (26.4	50 (35.5)		119 (84.4)	-	-	-
GS PE-unlikely	291 (54.5)	45 (15.5)	p < .001	263 (90.4)	7 (2.4)	18 (6.8)	11 (4.4)
GS PE-likely	243 (45.5)	78 (32.1)		208 (85.6)	-	-	-
GS PE-unlikely	302 (56.6)	51 (16.9)	p < .001	272 (90.0)	9 (3.0)	19 (7.0)	10 (4.0)
sGS PE-likely	232 (43.4)	72 (31.0)		199 (85.8)	-	-	-

[a] Significant differences were observed in the distribution of categories among all the scales (p < .001). [b] "%" corresponds to row percentages. [c] In the PE-unlikely group, aDD would not justify performing a CTCA. In the PE-likely group, DD tests were unjustified. [d]These values represent the number of CTCAs that would have been avoided if aDD was used instead of DD.(s)WS: (simplified) Wells' score. (s)GS: (simplified) revised Geneva Score. PE: pulmonary embolism. (a) DD: (age-adjusted) D-dimer. CTCA: Computed Tomography Chest Angiography

Table 3. Comparison of standard versus age-adjusted D-dimer

	Using standard D-dimer			Using age-adjusted D-dimer		
	Negative DD	**Positive DD**	**Total**	**Negative DD**	**Positive DD**	**Total**
No PE	13	340	353	31	323	353
PE	0	118	118	0	117	118
Total	13	458	471	31	440	471
Sensitivity: 100% Specificity: 3,7% Positive predictive value: 25,8% Negative predictive value: 100%				Sensitivity: 100% Specificity: 8,8% Positive predictive value: 26,6% Negative predictive value: 100%		

DD: D-dimer. PE: Pulmonary embolism

Table 4. Age distribution of comorbidities, risk factors, symptoms, final diagnosis and discharge destination

	Total N (%)	**<50 years N (%)**	**51-64 N (%)**	**65-74 N (%)**	**75-84 N (%)**	**85-89 N (%)**	**>90 years N (%)**	**P (linear)**	**<65 vs ≥65**	**PE vs no PE[a]**
PE frequency	123 (100)	12 (16.2)	24 (22.6)	25 (22.3)	33 (25.4)	18 (25.4)	11 (26.8)	0.710	0.33	-
Associated conditions										
Chronic kidney disease	36 (6.7)	1 (1.1)	1 (0.9)	8 (7.1)	15 (11.5)	5 (7)	6 (14.6)	**.007**	**.001**	.081
Heart failure	45 (8.4)	0 (0)	4 (3.8)	9 (8)	14 (10.8)	9 (12.7)	9 (22)	**.004**	**.002**	.647
COPD	89 (16.6)	1 (1.1)	23 (21.7)	26 (23.2)	27 (20.8)	9 (12.7)	3 (7.3)	**.003**	.315	**.023**
Cardiovascular risk factors										
Diabetes mellitus	159 (29.6)	17 (23)	29 (27.4)	35 (31.3)	39 (30)	24 (33.8)	15 (36.6)	.621	.096	**.005**
High blood pressure	292 (54.4)	42 (56.8)	59 (55.7)	68 (60.7)	68 (52.3)	36 (50.7)	19 (46.3)	.591	.814	.196
History of smoking	72 (13.4)	12 (16.2)	17 (16)	12 (10.7)	13 (10)	10 (14.1)	8 (19.5)	.486	.297	.654
Obesity	50 (9.3)	4 (5.4)	7 (6.6)	17 (15.2)	9 (6.9)	8 (11.3)	5 (12.2)	.136	**.045**	**.021**
Dyslipidemia	153 (28.5)	19 (25.7)	26 (24.5)	37 (33)	45 (34.6)	17 (23.9)	9 (22)	.288	.206	.956
Anticoagulatedz (Sintrom®)	51 (9.6)	3 (4.1)	8 (7.5)	10 (8.9)	15 (11.5)	9 (12.7)	6 (14.6)	.327	.112	.001
Oral contraceptives	6 (1.1)	5 (6.8)	1 (0.9)	0	0	0 (0)	0 (0)	**< .001**	**.001**	**.053**
Symptoms	**534**	74	106	112	130	71	41	-	-	
Dyspnea	367 (68.7)	53 (71.6)	76 (71.7)	74 (66.1)	88 (67.7)	46 (64.8)	30 (73.2)	.842	.479	.230
Cough	137 (25.7)	23 (31.1)	29 (27.4)	25 (29.1)	38 (29.2)	13 (18.31)	9 (22)	.549	.334	.547

Table 4. (Continued)

	Total N (%)	<50 years N (%)	51-64 N (%)	65-74 N (%)	75-84 N (%)	85-89 N (%)	>90 years N (%)	P (linear)	<65 vs ≥65	PE vs no PE[a]
Syncope	110 (20.6)	9 (12.2)	13 (12.3)	24 (21.4)	32 (24.6)	21 (29.6)	11 (27.6)	.067	**.004**	.175
Chest pain	195 (36.5)	42 (56.8)	40 (38.3)	52 (46.4)	38 (29.2)	16 (22.5)	7 (17.1)	<**.001**	**.002**	.194
Signs of DVT	57 (10.7)	7 (9.5)	8 (7.5)	9 (8.0)	19 (14.6)	7 (9.8)	7 (17.1)	.311	.153	.198
Hemoptysis	13 (2.4)	0 (0)	2 (1.9)	1 (0.9)	6 (4.6)	4 (5.6)	0 (0)	.082	.136	.316**
Discharge diagnosis										
Respiratory infection	90 (16.8)	12 (16.2)	16 (15.1)	23 (20.5)	24 (18.5)	7 (9.9)	8 (19.5)	.512	.933	.453
Heart failure	52 (9.7)	11 (14.9)	7 (6.6)	12 (10.7)	15 (11.5)	3 (4.2)	4 (9.8)	.265	.973	.302
Acute coronary syndrome	5 (0.9)	0 (0)	0 (0)	2 (1.8)	0 (0)	2 (2.8)	1 (2.4)	.186	.169	.871
Vasovagal syncope	36 (6.7)	4 (5.4)	5 (4.7)	11 (9.8)	8 (6.2)	8 (11.3)	0 (0)	.160	.200	.772
Others	176 (32.8)	17 (23)	38 (36)	33 (29.5)	47 (36.2)	29 (40.8)	12 (29.3)	.205	.406	.591
Combined	8 (1.5)	0 (0)	1 (0.9)	3 (2.7)	2 (1.5)	0 (0)	2 (4.9)	.247	.182	.119
Unknown ("dyspnea")	79 (14.7)	11 (14.9)	11 (10.4)	9 (8)	8 (6.2)	7 (9.9)	3 (7.3)	.432	.121	.060
Discharge destination										
To home	263 (49.3)	35 (47.3)	48 (45.3)	61 (54.5)	62 (47.7)	39 (54.9)	18 (43.9)	.622	.403	.176
Hospital admission	233 (43.6)	35 (50)	56 (54.7)	44 (41.9)	55 (45.4)	26 (42.2)	17 (48.8)	.444	.081	.139
Death	29 (5.4)	3 (0.6)	2 (0.4)	4 (0.7)	9 (1.7)	5 (0.9)	6 (1.1)	.05	.07	.699
Hospital transfer	9 (1.7)	1 (1.4)	0 (0)	3 (2.7)	4 (3.1)	1 (1.4)	0 (0)	.442	.132	.953

[a] Chi-squared test

Table 5. Cases of inadequate patient management according to each clinical probability score, and differences using age-adjusted D-dimer vs standard D-dimer values

	Total N (%)	**<50 years** N (%)	**51-64** N (%)	**65-74** N (%)	**75-84** N (%)	**85-89** N (%)	**>90 years** N (%)	**Linear P-value**
WS	83 (15.6)	18 (24.3)	21 (19.8)	12 (10.7)	13 (10.0)	2 (2.8)	7 (17.0)	<.001
sWS	128 (24.0)	26 (35.1)	31 (29.2)	25 (22.3)	29 (22.3)	8 (11.3)	8 (19.5)	<.001
GS	215 (40.3)	19 (25.7)	30 (28.3)	61 (54.5)	65 (50.0)	26 (36.6)	15 (36.6)	<.001
sGS	208 (39.0)	17 (23.0)	24 (22.64)	61 (54.5)	65 (50.0)	26 (36.6)	15 (36.6)	<.001
DD vs aDD (WS)	14 (2.6)	1 (1.4)	3 (2.8)	3 (2.7)	4 (3.1)	3 (4.2)	-	-

(s)WS: (simplified) Wells Score. (s)GS: (simplified) revised Geneva Score. (a)DD: (age-adjusted) D-dimer

Adequacy of Patient Management According to Age

Table 5 shows the number of cases in which serum DD tests or CTCA should not have been ordered according to each retrospective CPS, for each age group. Statistically significant differences were observed among all CPSs.

Discussion

In recent years, different studies analyzing the use of CPSs in suspected PE have reported significant differences in sociodemographic variables, PE prevalence and adherence to clinical guidelines. This has been linked to a number of internal and external factors (Booker & Johnson, 2017; Guijarro Merino et al., 2008), including selection and publication bias (Lucassen et al., 2011), differences in PE risk stratification, and patient variability (Ceriani et al., 2010). In our study, sociodemographic variables were similar to previous publications (Booker & Johnson, 2017; Lekerika et al., 2014; Lozano-Polo et al., 2018; Sanjuán et al., 2014). In the same vein, early mortality associated with PE (15.4%) was comparable to other reports (Uresandi et al., 2013), but higher than that observed in patients with normal blood pressure (Maestre Peiró et al., 2017). Notably, high variability in PE-related death reporting, owing to a lack of standardized definitions, has been emphasized in recent studies (Kraaijpoel et al., 2019).

The prevalence of PE (23.0%) was very similar to that described in other studies, mostly from Europe (Douma et al., 2011; Lozano-Polo et al., 2018; Marc Righini et al., 2014; Sanjuán et al., 2014) The proportion of subsegmental PEs found was also similar to that reported elsewhere (Carrier et al., 2010; Mountain et al., 2016). However, several publications, particularly from North America, reported a lower PE prevalence -closer to 10%- (Anjum et al., 2019; Booker & Johnson, 2017; Ceriani et al., 2010), which has been explained on the basis of CTCA overuse, defensive medicine, quick shift changeovers, and patients' demands (Booker & Johnson, 2017), among other factors. The marked difference in PE prevalence between North American and European studies is troublesome and could limit the validity of some CPSs since it is known that prevalence modifies the pre-test probability of a given disease (Chen et al., 2019; Lekerika et al., 2014; Lucassen et al., 2011). Lucassen et al. (Lucassen et al., 2011) suggest using CPSs with a higher sensitivity (i.e., sWS and GS) and gestalt assessment in settings with low PE prevalence. Righini et al. (M. Righini et al., 2019) emphasized that, in spite of its lower reproducibility, clinical assessment by expert clinicians to stratify the risk of PE is as feasible as the use of CPSs. In this context, Stüssi-Helbling et al. (Stüssi-Helbling et al., 2019) highlight that no CPS should replace proper clinical history taking, physical examination, or clinical information synthesis. A general recommendation –especially in physicians with limited clinical experience- is to use validated CPSs (Cronin & Dwamena, 2018; Uresandi et al., 2013), such as the WS.

The explicit use of CPSs (i.e., WS) observed in our study was only 15.2%, which is similar to other publications (Runyon et al., 2007; Sanjuán et al., 2014). After retrospective WS calculation, less than 10% of these cases were classified into a different category, which can be interpreted as an indirect measurement of the bias due to retrospective scale reconstruction. Despite the low explicit use of WS, almost 90% of the serum DD tests ordered were justified according to the retrospective WS. This trend was also observed in the rest of the CPSs (84.4-90.4%). We hypothesize two possible explanations for these findings. On the one hand, they could be due to an implicit use of CPSs by clinicians. However, it seems unlikely that they did not annotate the score in the electronic record of the episode. On the other hand, they could be explained by the fact that gestalt assessment is used to estimate the risk of PE instead of CPSs. In our opinion, this assumption seems more likely, but it should be confirmed in future studies.

Differences in risk stratification among CPSs are relevant, considering that the predictive value of CTCA varies depending on the risk of PE (Moores et al., 2016; Stein et al., 2006) and that heparin is indicated in patients with high risk of PE (Lekerika et al., 2014; Uresandi et al., 2013). In the present study, PE prevalence in both PE-likely and PE-unlikely groups significantly differed among CPSs. In a recent systematic review, Ceriani et al. (Ceriani et al., 2010) found that the prevalence of PE in European countries was 11.5% in PE-unlikely and 36.7% in PE-likely categories, while these percentages were 6.5% and 32.9%, respectively, in the United States. Analogously, Van der Pol et al. (van der Pol et al., 2018) reported a PE prevalence of 15% and 42% in PE-unlikely and PE-likely categories, respectively. In our study, PE prevalence in the former group was 15-21%, and 32-36% in the latter, according to the WS and GS. These rates are very similar to those reported by Gibson et al. according to the sWS (Gibson et al., 2008). In summary, while the observed prevalence of PE in the PE-likely category was similar to that reported in other European studies, we found a significantly higher PE prevalence in the PE-likely group.

Regarding the use and validity of the serum DD tests, aDD has demonstrated to increase the negative predictive value of standard DD by 12-24% (Lozano-Polo et al., 2018; Marc Righini et al., 2014). Moreover, guideline adherence increases by 7.6% when aDD is combined with the sWS (Lozano-Polo et al., 2018). Our results are consistent with these data, although the increase in overall specificity was not that high (i.e., 5.1%), and guideline adherence (i.e., adequacy of patient management) slightly improved (by 2.6%). Therefore, although current international guidelines accept both DD and aDD values (Konstantinides et al., 2019), our results support the use of the latter.

Concerning retrospective CPSs, patient management adequacy was superior to 85% according to the WS, although this percentage decreased to 75% in sWS, and was around 60% in GS and sGS. These differences could be explained by the item "another diagnosis is less likely than PE", which substantially influences test positivity and, thus, its sensitivity and specificity (Lucassen et al., 2011). Under the assumption that these percentages may reflect adherence to clinical guidelines, they are significantly higher than those reported by other authors. For example, Lozano-Polo et al. (Lozano-Polo et al., 2018) reported guideline adherence of 39.2% and 53.2% according to the GS and WS, respectively. Similar proportions were reported by Sanjuan et al. (45,8%) (Sanjuán et al., 2014) and by Molaee et al. (43,9%) (Molaee et al., 2015). Furthermore, we observed significant differences in guideline adherence between age groups, although not so notable as in other studies (Lozano-Polo et al., 2018).

This study presents some limitations. First, the retrospective calculation of CPSs may entail some biases, e.g., increasing the likelihood of positively scoring the item "another diagnosis is less likely than PE". Second, the use of two-level scores could entail some differences in comparison with three-level scores, despite both proved to have a similar yield (Douma et al., 2011). Third, our results are not directly comparable to studies analyzing all cases suspicious of PE regardless of whether or not they underwent CTCA, since we only included those patients in whom a CTCA was performed to rule out PE. Finally, the fact that the period of study covered 1 year, and that it was performed in a single institution limits the generalizability of our findings.

Conclusion

Our results confirm the trend observed in other studies regarding the low explicit use of WS in the ED. Nevertheless, based on the retrospective calculation of the WS in our study, this does not necessarily imply that the management of patients with suspected PE is completely inadequate. Moreover, the similar rate of positive CTCAs, as compared to other geographically related studies, might be explained by the fact that gestalt assessment shows a similar yield compared to the use of CPSs. Our results need further validation through analytical studies with appropriate prospective designs.

References

Alfonso Figueredo, E., Pérez Alvarez, M. L., Reyes Sanamé, F. A., Batista Acosta, Y., & Peña Garcell, Y. (2016). Nuevas consideraciones en el tratamiento del tromboembolismo pulmonar [*New considerations in the treatment of pulmonary thromboembolism*]. *Revista Cubana de Medicina*, *55*(3), 224–238.

Anjum, O., Bleeker, H., & Ohle, R. (2019). Computed tomography for suspected pulmonary embolism results in a large number of non-significant incidental findings and follow-up investigations. *Emergency Radiology*, *26*(1), 29–35. https://doi.org/10.1007/s10140-018-1641-8.

Booker, M. T., & Johnson, J. O. (2017). Optimizing CT Pulmonary Angiogram Utilization in a Community Emergency Department: A Pre- and Postintervention Study. *Journal of the American College of Radiology*, *14*(1), 65–71. https://doi.org/10.1016/j.jacr.2016.08.007.

Carrier, M., Righini, M., Wells, P. S., Perrier, A., Anderson, D. R., Rodger, M. A., Pleasance, S., & Le Gal, G. (2010). Subsegmental pulmonary embolism diagnosed by computed tomography: incidence and clinical implications. A systematic review and meta-analysis of the management outcome studies. *Journal of Thrombosis and Haemostasis*, *8*(8), 1716–1722. https://doi.org/10.1111/j.1538-7836.2010.03938.x.

Ceriani, E., Combescure, C., Le Gal, G., Nendaz, M., Perneger, T., Bounameaux, H., Perrier, A., & Righini, M. (2010). Clinical prediction rules for pulmonary embolism: a systematic review and meta-analysis. *Journal of Thrombosis and Haemostasis*, *8*(5), 957–970. https://doi.org/10.1111/j.1538-7836.2010.03801.x.

Chen, Z., Deblois, S., Toporowicz, K., Boldeanu, I., Francoeur, M.-O., Sadouni, M., Lepanto, L., & Chartrand-Lefebvre, C. (2019). Yield of CT pulmonary angiography in the diagnosis of acute pulmonary embolism: short report. *BMC Research Notes*, *12*(1), 41. https://doi.org/10.1186/s13104-019-4076-8.

Cronin, P., & Dwamena, B. A. (2018). A Clinically Meaningful Interpretation of the Prospective Investigation of Pulmonary Embolism Diagnosis (PIOPED) II and III

Data. *Academic Radiology*, *25*(5), 561–572. https://doi.org/10.1016/j.acra.2017.11.014.

Douma, R. A., Mos, I. C. M., Erkens, P. M. G., Nizet, T. A. C., Durian, M. F., Hovens, M. M., van Houten, A. A., Hofstee, H. M. A., Klok, F. A., ten Cate, H., Ullmann, E. F., Büller, H. R., Kamphuisen, P. W., & Huisman, M. V. (2011). Performance of 4 clinical decision rules in the diagnostic management of acute pulmonary embolism: A prospective cohort study. *Annals of Internal Medicine*, *154*(11), 709–718. https://doi.org/10.7326/0003-4819-154-11-201106070-00002.

Gibson, N. S., Sohne, M., Kruip, M. J. H. A., Tick, L. W., Gerdes, V. E., Bossuyt, P. M., Wells, P. S., Buller, H. R., & Christopher study investigators. (2008). Further validation and simplification of the Wells clinical decision rule in pulmonary embolism. *Thrombosis and Haemostasis*, *99*(01), 229–234. https://doi.org/10.1160/TH07-05-0321.

Guijarro Merino, R., Montes Santiago, J., & San Román Terán, C. M. (2008). Epidemiología hospitalaria de la enfermedad tromboembólica venosa en España [*Hospital epidemiology of venous thromboembolic disease in Spain*]. *Medicina Clinica*, *131*(SUPPL. 2), 2–9. https://doi.org/10.1016/S0025-7753(08) 76442-X.

Jiménez, D., de Miguel-Díez, J., Guijarro, R., Trujillo-Santos, J., Otero, R., Barba, R., Muriel, A., Meyer, G., Yusen, R. D., & Monreal, M. (2016). Trends in the Management and Outcomes of Acute Pulmonary Embolism: Analysis From the RIETE Registry. *Journal of the American College of Cardiology*, *67*(2), 162–170. https://doi.org/10.1016/J.JACC.2015.10.060.

Konstantinides, S. V, Meyer, G., Becattini, C., Bueno, H., Geersing, G.-J., Harjola, V.-P., Huisman, M. V, Humbert, M., Jennings, C. S., Jiménez, D., Kucher, N., Lang, I. M., Lankeit, M., Lorusso, R., Mazzolai, L., Meneveau, N., Ní Áinle, F., Prandoni, P., Pruszczyk, P., … Pepke-Zaba, J. (2019). 2019 ESC Guidelines for the diagnosis and management of acute pulmonary embolism developed in collaboration with the European Respiratory Society (ERS). *European Heart Journal*. https://doi.org/10.1093/eurheartj/ehz405.

Kraaijpoel, N., Tritschler, T., Guillo, E., Girard, P., & Le Gal, G. (2019). Definitions, adjudication, and reporting of pulmonary embolism–related death in clinical studies: A systematic review. *Journal of Thrombosis and Haemostasis*, *17*(10), 1590–1607. https://doi.org/10.1111/jth.14570.

Lekerika, N., Arana-Arri, E., García Montero, A., García, L., Gómez, A., & Carreras, M. (2014). Probabilidad clínica de tromboembolismo pulmonar: beneficio diagnóstico de las escalas de predicción y de los dímeros D [*Clinical probability of pulmonary thromboembolism: diagnostic benefit of prediction scales and D-dimers*]. *Emergencias*, *26*, 243–250.

Lozano-Polo, L., Puig-Campmany, M., Herrera-Mateo, S., Mateo-Roca, M., Santos-Rodríguez, J. A., & Benito-Vales, S. (2018). Diagnóstico en urgencias del embolismo pulmonar en ancianos : adherencia a las guías y valor del dímero-D corregido por edad [*Emergency diagnosis of pulmonary embolism in the elderly: adherence to guidelines and age-corrected D-dimer value*]. *Emergencias*, *30*, 321–327.

Lucassen, W., Geersing, G.-J., Erkens, P. M. G., Reitsma, J. B., Moons, K. G. M., Büller, H., & van Weert, H. C. (2011). Clinical Decision Rules for Excluding Pulmonary Embolism: A Meta-analysis. *Annals of Internal Medicine*, *155*(7), 448. https://doi.org/10.7326/0003-4819-155-7-201110040-00007.

Maestre Peiró, A., Gonzálvez Gasch, A., & Monreal Bosch, M. (2017). Actualización en la estratificación de riesgo del tromboembolismo pulmonar agudo sintomático [*Update on risk stratification of symptomatic acute pulmonary thromboembolism*]. *Revista Clinica Espanola*, *217*(6), 342–350. https://doi.org/10.1016/j.rce.2017.02.018.

Molaee, S., Ghanaati, H., Safavi, E., Foroumandi, M., & Peiman, S. (2015). Computed Tomography Pulmonary Angiography for Evaluation of Patients With Suspected Pulmonary Embolism: Use or Overuse. *Iranian Journal of Radiology: A Quarterly Journal Published by the Iranian Radiological Society*, *12*(3), e22383. https://doi.org/10.5812/iranjradiol.12(2)2015.22383.

Moores, L., Kline, J., Portillo, A. K., Resano, S., Vicente, A., Arrieta, P., Corres, J., Tapson, V., Yusen, R. D., & Jiménez, D. (2016). Multidetector computed tomographic pulmonary angiography in patients with a high clinical probability of pulmonary embolism. *Journal of Thrombosis and Haemostasis*, *14*(1), 114–120. https://doi.org/10.1111/jth.13188.

Mountain, D., Keijzers, G., Chu, K., Joseph, A., Read, C., Blecher, G., Furyk, J., Bharat, C., Velusamy, K., Munro, A., Baker, K., Kinnear, F., Mukherjee, A., Watkins, G., Buntine, P., Livesay, G., & Fatovich, D. (2016). RESPECT-ED: Rates of Pulmonary Emboli (PE) and Sub-Segmental PE with Modern Computed Tomographic Pulmonary Angiograms in Emergency Departments: A Multi-Center Observational Study Finds Significant Yield Variation, Uncorrelated with Use or Small PE Rates. *PLOS ONE*, *11*(12), e0166483. https://doi.org/10.1371/journal.pone.0166483.

Raja, A. S., Greenberg, J. O., Qaseem, A., Denberg, T. D., Fitterman, N., & Schuur, J. D. (2015). Evaluation of patients with suspected acute pulmonary embolism: Best practice advice from the Clinical Guidelines Committee of the American College of Physicians. *Annals of Internal Medicine*, *163*(9), 701–711. https://doi.org/10.7326/M14-1772.

Righini, M., Robert-Ebadi, H., & Le Gal, G. (2019). Diagnostic de l'embolie pulmonaire [*Diagnosis of pulmonary embolism*]. *La Revue de Médecine Interne*, *40*(7), 440–444. https://doi.org/10.1016/j.revmed.2 019.01.004.

Righini, Marc, Van Es, J., Den Exter, P. L., Roy, P. M., Verschuren, F., Ghuysen, A., Rutschmann, O. T., Sanchez, O., Jaffrelot, M., Trinh-Duc, A., Le Gall, C., Moustafa, F., Principe, A., Van Houten, A. A., Ten Wolde, M., Douma, R. A., Hazelaar, G., Erkens, P. M. G., Van Kralingen, K. W., … Le Gal, G. (2014). Age-adjusted D-dimer cutoff levels to rule out pulmonary embolism: The ADJUST-PE study. *JAMA - Journal of the American Medical Association*, *311*(11), 1117–1124. https://doi.org/10.1001/jama.2014.2135.

Runyon, M. S., Richman, P. B., & Kline, J. A. (2007). Emergency Medicine Practitioner Knowledge and Use of Decision Rules for the Evaluation of Patients with Suspected Pulmonary Embolism: Variations by Practice Setting and Training Level. *Academic Emergency Medicine*, *14*(1), 53–57. https://doi.org/10.1197/j.aem.2006.07.032

Sandoval B., J., & Florenzano V., M. (2015). Diagnóstico Y Tratamiento Del Tromboembolismo Pulmonar [*Diagnosis and treatment of pulmonary thromboembolism*]. *Revista Médica Clínica Las Condes*, *26*(3), 338–343. https://doi.org/10.1016/j.rmclc.2015.04.021.

Sanjuán, P., Rodríguez-Núñez, N., Rábade, C., Lama, A., Ferreiro, L., González-Barcala, F. J., Álvarez-Dobaño, J. M., Toubes, M. E., Golpe, A., & Valdés, L. (2014). Escalas de probabilidad clínica y algoritmo diagnóstico en la embolia pulmonar: ¿se siguen en la práctica clínica? [*Clinical probability scales and diagnostic algorithm in pulmonary embolism: are they followed in clinical practice?*] *Archivos de Bronconeumologia*, *50*(5), 172–178. https://doi.org/10.1016/j.arbr.2014.03.013.

Stein, P. D., Fowler, S. E., Goodman, L. R., Gottschalk, A., Hales, C. A., Hull, R. D., Leeper, K. V., Popovich, J., Quinn, D. A., Sos, T. A., Sostman, H. D., Tapson, V. F., Wakefield, T. W., Weg, J. G., Woodard, P. K., & PIOPED II Investigators. (2006). Multidetector Computed Tomography for Acute Pulmonary Embolism. *New England Journal of Medicine*, *354*(22), 2317–2327. https://doi.org/10.1056/NEJMoa052367.

Stüssi-Helbling, M., Arrigo, M., & Huber, L. C. (2019). Pearls and Myths in the Evaluation of Patients with Suspected Acute Pulmonary Embolism. *The American Journal of Medicine*, *132*(6), 685–691. https://doi.org/10.1016/j.amjmed.2019.01.011.

Tritschler, T., Kraaijpoel, N., Le Gal, G., & Wells, P. S. (2018). Venous Thromboembolism. *JAMA*, *320*(15), 1583–1594. https://doi.org/10.1016/B978-0-12-803678-5.00506-3.

Uresandi, F., Monreal, M., García-Bragado, F., Domenech, P., Lecumberri, R., Escribano, P., Zamorano, J. L., Jiménez, S., Ruiz-Artacho, P., Lozano, F., Romera, A., & Jiménez, D. (2013). Consenso nacional sobre el diagnóstico, estratificación de riesgo y tratamiento de los pacientes con tromboembolia pulmonar [*National consensus on the diagnosis, risk stratification and treatment of patients with pulmonary thromboembolism*]. *Archivos de Bronconeumología*, *49*(12), 534–547. https://doi.org/10.1016/j.arbres.2013.07.008.

van der Pol, L. M., Bistervels, I. M., van Mens, T. E., van der Hulle, T., Beenen, L. F. M., den Exter, P. L., Kroft, L. J. M., Mairuhu, A. T. A., Middeldorp, S., van Werkhoven, J. M., ten Wolde, M., Huisman, M. V., & Klok, F. A. (2018). Lower prevalence of subsegmental pulmonary embolism after application of the YEARS diagnostic algorithm. *British Journal of Haematology*, *183*(4), 629–635. https://doi.org/10.1111/bjh.15556.

Van Es, N. (2017). The original and simplified Wells rules and age-adjusted D-dimer testing to rule out pulmonary embolism: an individual patient data meta-analysis. *Journal of Thrombosis and Haemostasis*, *15*, 678–684. https://doi.org/10.1111/jth.13630.

Chapter 4

Efficacy and Security of Ultrasound-Assisted Catheter-Directed Thrombolysis in Acute Pulmonary Embolism: A Systematic Review

M. Crespo Balbuena[1,2], MD
and Antonio Jesús Láinez Ramos-Bossini[1,2,3], MD
[1]Department of Radiology,
Hospital Universitario Virgen de las Nieves, Granada, Spain
[2]Biosanitary Research Institute, Granada, Spain
[3]Department of Psychiatry, School of Medicine,
University of Granada, Granada, Spain

Abstract

Traditionally, acute pulmonary embolism (PE) has been treated with anticoagulation and/or systemic thrombolysis. However, in recent years improvements in interventional therapeutic techniques have facilitated the management of numerous pathologies where conventional therapies are contraindicated or not free of considerable complications. Mechanical or pharmaco-mechanical thrombolysis directed by percutaneous catheter is one of the options available for the treatment of PE and its application is increasing in the emergency department. Ultrasound-assisted catheter-directed thrombolysis (USACDT) is one of the most recently-implemented techniques. The aim of this study is to evaluate the efficacy and safety of USACDT for the treatment of PE according to the evidence available to date.

We conducted a systematic review by searching the main medical databases. We prioritized the inclusion of experimental and observational studies. We also reviewed clinical practice guidelines. We discuss the different aspects related on the topic according to the available literature.

In: Understanding and Treating Acute Pulmonary Embolism
Editor: James K. Edwards
ISBN: 979-8-88697-149-1

Current evidence reveals that USACDT is a feasible treatment for PE that reduced mean pulmonary artery pressure and other functional variables, with low risk of major bleeding. Further research is required to determine the most appropriate indications of this treatment.

Keywords: pulmonary embolism, ultrasound-assisted catheter-directed thrombolysis, computed tomography

Introduction

Pulmonary embolism (PE) is the third leading cause of cardiovascular mortality [1]. Traditionally, PE has been treated with anticoagulation and/or systemic thrombolysis. In recent years, this conventional approach has changed with the development of new endovascular technologies. Due to the wide range of therapeutic options, the concept of the PE response team (PERT) has emerged [2]. One of the most important goals of the PERT Clinical Practice and Protocol Development Committee is to characterize consensus practice actions for clinical care [3].

According to the PERT guidelines, after the diagnosis of PE, risk stratification is necessary [3]. The most commonly used categories are: massive or high-risk, submassive or intermediate-risk, and low risk, as proposed by the American Heart Association (AHA) [4] and the European Society of Cardiology (ESC) [5], respectively.

Risk stratification is based primarily on two factors. On the one hand, the difficulty of the right ventricle (RV) to overcome the afterload caused by the thrombi present in the pulmonary arteries (i.e., right heart straing). On the other hand, the presence or absence of hypotension defined as a systolic blood pressure [SBP] <90 mmHg for more than 15 minutes, a decrease in SBP of 40 mmHg or more from baseline, or the need for hemodynamic support. When both parameters are present, PE is stratified as high-risk, while in the absence of hypotension, it is categorized as intermediate-risk [4-5]. In the latter group, additional stratification can be performed based on biomarkers, imaging examinations and other clinical data described by the AHA and ESC, so that intermediate-high-risk PE is also possible [5]. This may help to gauge the risk of hemodynamic decompensation and suggest the need for more aggressive treatment, considering that patients with RV dysfunction and abnormal biomarkers have higher mortality risk [6].

The severity of PE determines the therapeutic strategy to be performed. Accordingly, low-risk PE is treated with anticoagulation drugs, while the therapeutic approach in high-risk PE is systemic fibrinolysis except in cases of contraindication. In the latter case, surgical thrombectomy or catheter-guided mechanical thrombectomy may be considered depending on availability [3, 5]. In-hospital mortality attributable to PE has been found to be lower in unstable patients who received thrombolytic therapy compared to those who did not [7].

The management of intermediate-risk PE is more controversial, as the risk of life-threatening bleeding complications seems too high for the expected benefits of this treatment [8]. Nevertheless, early resolution of pulmonary obstruction leads to a rapid reduction in pulmonary artery pressure and resistance, with a concomitant improvement in RV function [9]. Furthermore, in a randomized comparative study of heparin vs. alteplase in normotensive patients with acute PE and evidence of RV dysfunction or pulmonary hypertension (i.e., intermediate-risk PE) thrombolytic therapy reduced the incidence of escalation in PE severity, with no changes in mortality [10]. Subsequently, the PEITHO clinical trial [8] showed a decrease in all-cause mortality in the tenecteplase-treated group versus the control group, although an increase in major hemorrhagic and intracranial complications was observed. Therefore, for intermediate-risk PE, the most updated guidelines recommend anticoagulation and close monitoring [3, 5] due to the risk of hemodynamic decompensation. In the case of intermediate-high-risk PE, the use of reduced doses of fibrinolysis, surgical thrombectomy or catheter-guided mechanical thrombectomy is recommended depending on availability [3, 5].

The use of "ultrasound-assisted catheter-directed thrombolysis" (USACDT) makes it possible to mechanically dissolve the thrombi directly in the pulmonary arteries, reducing the dose of fibrinolytic agents. For instance, the EkoSonic (EKOS/BTG, Bothell, Washington) USACDT system consists of a conventional infusion catheter containing an inner wire that transmits high frequency, low power ultrasound waves to improve penetration of the thrombolytic agent at the site of action [3]. Recent meta-analyses published between 2018-2020- advocate promising results [11-14] and raise the need for further studies [11, 14]. Considering the novelty and potential impact of USACDT in the treatment of PE, the aim of this study is to evaluate its efficacy and safety according to the evidence available to date.

Methods

Eligibility Criteria

The systematic review design and selection criteria were based on the PICO search strategy. The population consisted of patients with PE treated with USACDT (i.e., intervention) and in whom the efficacy or safety (i.e., outcomes) of the procedure was evaluated, either alone or in comparison with another treatment (i.e., comparison). The Preferred Reporting Items for Systematic Reviews and Meta-Analyses (PRISMA) guidelines were followed.

Accordingly, the inclusion criteria were as follows: clinical trials, prospective and retrospective observational studies published as original articles on the use of USACDT in patients with PE that included quantitative results on at least one of the primary outcomes (see 'variables' subsection). Exclusion criteria were reviews, systematic reviews, case reports, letters, and other study designs.

Information Sources and Search Strategy

Two authors searched the PubMed database. Different search strategies were used to optimize the number of relevant outcomes, including keywords such as "pulmonary embolism" and "ultrasound-assisted," "ultrasound-accelerated" or "ultrasound-facilitated," using several combinations to increase the sensitivity of the search.

The final search was "pulmonary embolism" AND ("Ultrasound-assisted catheter-directed thrombolysis" OR "Ultrasound-assisted thrombolysis" OR "ultrasound facilitated" OR "ultrasound-accelerated thrombolysis" OR "sonolysis" OR "sonothrombolysis" OR "EKOS"). The following filters were used: abstract and full text available since January 1, 2020. No language restriction was established. The search was updated to March 24, 2022.

First, all titles and abstracts of interest were reviewed and those that were not the subject of the current review were excluded. Second, those which did not meet the eligibility criteria were excluded. Finally, the screened studies were fully read to assess whether they met all eligibility criteria or not. Figure 1 shows the flow diagram of the study.

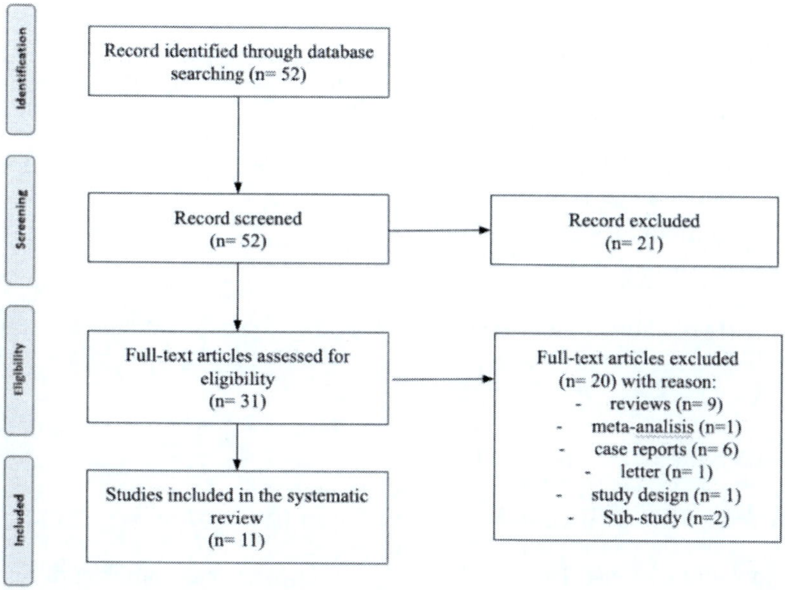

Figure 1. Flow diagram depicting the search conducted in this review.

Variables and Data Extraction

The variables in the review were classified into measures of efficacy and safety assessment and grouped according to the type of study (clinical trial or observational study) into outcomes related to treatment efficacy and outcomes related to treatment safety. The former included quantitative measures of:

- The variation in RV overload (i.e., right heart strain) due to the effect of treatment.
- The reduction of pulmonary artery pressure due to treatment effect.

Regarding the second group, it must be noted that there are variations in the classification of bleeding among different studies. The BARC (Bleeding Academic Research Consortium) scale, the International Society of Thrombosis and Haemostasis (ISTH) and the Global Utilization of Streptokinase and TPA For Occluded Arteries definition for bleeding (GUSTO) bleeding criteria are used indistinctly. We tried to homogenize the results by considering the criteria of these scales. Accordingly, complications occurring during hospitalization were grouped as follows:

- Major bleeding event
- Minor bleeding event
- Intracraneal hemorrhage
- Hemodynamic instability
- In-hospital death

The two authors of the work independently extracted data from the selected articles and reviewed them together to resolve discrepancies.

Results and Discussion

Characteristics of the Articles Included in the Review

A total of 11 articles were finally included in the review after applying the inclusion and exclusion criteria. Nine of them were retrospective observational studies, of which 2 were multicenter, 1 prospective single-center observational, and 1 randomized controlled trial. They are shown in Table 1, identified by the surname of the first author and the year of publication. Although 63.6% of the studies were from the United States, there are representative articles from Europe and Asia. All studies reported quantitative data on the efficacy or safety of USACDT in terms of changes in RV and pulmonary artery pressure or in terms of the number of complications during hospitalization for this procedure. The characteristics of the patients included in each study who were treated with USACDT are listed in Table 2.

Outcomes Related to Treatment Efficacy

Of the 10 observational studies included in the review, 5 (50%) provide quantitative data on the decrease in RV overload expressed as the difference in RV/LV ratio before (pre-) and after (post-) intervention, being statistically significant in all cases.

Regarding the decrease in pulmonary artery pressure, 4 (40%) studies allowed us to extract quantitative data and there is also a statistically significant difference in favor of treatment with USACDT. Table 3 shows the results of the retrospective or prospective observational studies included in the review.

Table 1. Main characteristics of the studies included in the review

	Study	Journal	Country	Study design	Aim
1	Klein 2022 [15]	Can Respir J.	Germany	Retrospective observational study, single-center	To evaluate the safety and efficiency of UACDT in patients with intermediate-high-risk or high-risk PE.
2	Robles 2022 [16]	Innovations (Phila).	EEUU	Retrospective observational study, single-center	To evaluate the long-term efficacy and safety of EKOS in submassive PE.
3	Jiang 2021 [17]	Cureus	United States	Retrospective observational study, multi-center	To determine clinical outcomes for a population of patients with intermediate-risk PE receiving anticoagulation with and without thrombolytic therapy.
4	Avgerinos 2021 [18]	JACC Cardiovasc Interv.	United States	Randomized controlled trial.	To determine whether ultrasound-assisted thrombolysis (USAT) is superior to standard catheter-directed thrombolysis (SCDT) in pulmonary arterial thrombus reduction for patients with submassive pulmonary embolism (sPE).
5	Stępniewski 2021 [19]	Am J Cardiol.	United States	Prospective observational study, single-center.	To investigate changes in invasive pulmonary hemodynamics during very low-alteplase-dose USAT of 10 mg administered within reduced 5-hour infusion in patients with intermediate-to-high-risk PE.
6	Kline 2021 [20]	J Thromb Thrombolysis.	United States	Retrospective observational study, single-center	To compare the efficacy and safety of catheter-directed USAT versus systemic anticoagulation alone in submassive PE.
7	Wang 2020 [21]	Acta Cardiol Sin.	China	Retrospective Observational Study, single-center.	To determine clinical outcomes of USACDT in treating intermediate-to-high-risk PE.
8	Saylan 2020 [22]	Turk Gogus Kalp Damar Cerrahisi Derg.	Turkey	Retrospective Observational Study, single-center	To evaluate the efficacy and the safety of the EkoSonicTM endovascular system applications in patients hospitalized with the diagnosis of intermediate-high-risk PE.

Table 1. (Continued)

	Study	Journal	Country	Study design	Aim
9	Wayne 2020 [23]	J Thromb Thrombolysis.	United States	Retrospective observational study, single-center.	To evaluate the implementation at our institution of shorter duration (4 h) of USACDT and lower dosing strategy (tPA 1 mg/h) administered with USACDT to patient with PE.
10	Beyer 2020 [24]	Chest.	United States	Retrospective observational study, multi-center.	To examine practice patterns of systemic thrombolysis and catheter-directed thrombolysis (CDT) and to compare outcomes after CDT with ultrasound facilitation (CDT-US) and CDT alone.
11	Hooks 2020 [25]	Vasc Endovascular Surg.	United States	Retrospective observational study, single-center.	To assess outcome mea-sures at a community-based hospital systems and compared results to known studies.

Table 2. Main characteristics of the patients included in the studies reviewed

	Study	n (M/F)	Age. Mean ± SD	Body mass index (kg/m²)	Risk	Alteplase dose (mg)	Fibrinolysis time (h)
1	Klein 2022	51(21/30)	63 ± 18	31.1 ± 7.1	I-R* H-R	11.5	15
2	Robles 2022	26(11/15)	59	37	I-R*	23	12
3	Jiang 2021	47(17/20)	59.4 ±15.1	-	I-R*	22.8 + 6.8	12.7 + 3.0
4	Avgerinos 2021	40(23/17)	52 ± 13	37 ± 8	I-R*	19 ± 7	14 ± 6
5	Stępniewski 2021	12(7/5)	64	-	I-R*	10	5
6	Kline 2021	40(20/20)	58 (19 –81)	31.1 (19.3 –70.5)	I-R*	23.5 mg	13
7	Wang 2020	42(18/24	58.93 ± 20.48	25.53 ± 4.42	I-R* H-R	44.54 ± 20.55	39.14 ± 19.06
8	Saylan 2020	15(7/8)	64.7±17.8	-	I-R*	-	-
9	Wayne 2020	31(10/21)	49.0 (14.3)	37.3 (8.8)	I-R H-R	Different dose/time strategies	-
10	Beyer 2020	417(198/219)	59.8 ± 15.3	-	-	-	-
11	Hooks 2020	83(41/42)	59.9 + 13.5	34.8 + 7.7	I-R* H-R	24mg	12 o 24h

*Patients included in these studies with a diagnosis of Intermediate-Risk PE meet the sub-stratification criteria for Intermediate-High-Risk PE of the AHA or ESC [3-5].

Table 3. Main results of the retrospective or prospective observational studies included in the review

Study	Median RV/LV ratio pre-USACDT/ post-USACDT	p	Mean sPAP (mmHg) pre-USACDT/ post-USACDT	p
Klein 2022	from 1.13 to 0.96	<0.001	from 47 to 32	<0.0002
Robles 2022	from 1.47 to 0.91	<0.05	-	-
Jiang 2021	no data available	-		-
Stępniewski 2021	from 1.44 to 0.98	0.003	from 53 to 37.5	0.02
Kline 2021	no data available	-		-
Wang 2020	from 1.46 to 0.79	< 0.01	from 60.77 to 41.95	<0.01
Saylan 2020	from 42.4 to 37.3 ± 4.1	0.001	from 44 to 36**	0.001
Wayne 2020	no data available	-		-
Beyer 2020	no data available	-		-
Hooks 2020	no data available	-		-

*Diameter in millimeters of the RV, pre-USACDT and post-USACDT.

**Mean pulmonary artery pressure.

Regarding the randomized controlled clinical trial included in the review (Avgerinos 2021) the USACDT-treated group experienced a reduction in the RV/LV ratio from 1.54 ± 0.3 to 0.37 ± 0.34 at 48 hours after the intervention; and showed a reduction in mean pulmonary artery pressure from 31 ± 4 to 22 ± 7 after USACDT (P < 0.001) [18].

Outcomes Related to Treatment Safety

Complications during admission after the procedure were diverse and very different in frequency, with varied clinical significance, including technical problems with the catheter ultrasound probe, vasovagal symptoms, or hematomas at the puncture site [15] or in the pulmonary artery [22]. In addition, different criteria were used to establish the severity of bleeding: BARC scale [15, 23, International Society of Thrombosis and Hemostasis (ISTH) [16, 17, 19, 20]; the GUSTO bleeding criteria [21, 22, 25], although they all differentiate between major and minor bleeding. The results are shown in Table 4.

As for the randomized controlled clinical trial included in the review - Avgerinos 2021 - in the group treated with USCDT, 2 major bleedings were documented (1 stroke and 1 vaginal bleed requiring transfusion) [18].

Table 4. Observational studies. Complications during admission

	Klein 2022 (n = 51)	Robles 2022 (n = 26)	Jiang 2021 (n = 47)	Stępniewski 2021 (n = 12)	Kline 2021 (n = 40)	Wang 2020 (n = 42)	Saylan 2020 (n = 15)	Wayne 2020 (n = 31)	Beyer 2020 (n = 417)	Hooks 2020 (n = 83)
Major bleeding event	6	1	2	0	0	9	0	3	41***	1
Minor bleeding event	4	-	1	1	6	18	1**	8	-	4
Intracraneal hemorrhage	0	0	1	0	0	1	0	0	<10	0
Hemodynamic instability	0	-	1	0	0	*	0	6	<10	-
In-hospital death	2!	0	0	0	0	3 (< 30 días)	0	1	17	1
Total (%)	23.5	3.8	10.6	8.3	15	73.8	6.6	58	13.9	7.2

*Specifies that 8 of the major bleedings were accompanied by hemodynamic instability.

**Pulmonary hematoma.

*** Includes intracranial hemorrhages but does not specify how many.

Discussion

In this review we present the data published from January 2020 to March 2022 in experimental and observational prospective and retrospective analytical studies on the efficacy and safety of USACDT in the treatment of PE. The results are heterogeneous; most of the studies are observational (and retrospective) and only one randomized controlled clinical trial is available to date. Regarding the population included in the studies, the mean age is generally in the 6th-7th decade of life and in 10 of the 11 articles the patients presented at least one intermediate-high-risk PE.

According to the available evidence, there is insufficient data on the value of USACDT as a preventive measure in intermediate-high-risk PE. For instance, in a patient with signs of RV overload without other signs of severity or imminent hemodynamic instability -which would make the PE to be stratified as intermediate-high-risk- management should be anticoagulation alone. However, it has been shown that rapid resolution of the obstruction leads to a rapid reduction in pulmonary resistance and consequently improves RV function (9), so that more studies are needed in these patients.

The variables referred to in the articles for the assessment of the efficacy and safety of USACDT in PE are diverse. For the measurement of efficacy, the most commonly used variables are the difference in the RV/LV ratio and pulmonary artery pressure after treatment It is not clear which one may be more useful, since both have their advantages and disadvantages. First, the RV/LV ratio is an operator-dependent measurement, whether measured by echocardiography or by CT angiography. However, it is a non-invasive measurement and can be calculated in retrospective studies in which there are pre- and post-treatment CT angiography scans. In contrast, the measurement of pulmonary pressures is an invasive procedure, although less variable between observers. Regarding the data collected, 6 of the 11 publications provide quantitative results on the difference in these variables before and after the intervention, with a statistically significant difference in all cases, both in the RV/LV ratio and in the decrease in pulmonary artery pressure. In other words, the results are similar to the latest meta-analyses published between 2018-2020 [11-14], in which USACDT was shown to be an effective procedure associated with significant hemodynamic and clinical improvement in patients with massive and submassive PE.

Regarding treatment safety, the available data are more heterogeneous. First, there are variations in the collection of results using different scales in the qualification of bleeding, although they all differentiate between major and minor bleeding events. Second, the qualification of complications in general is different in each study, since some even refer to vasovagal syncope [15], while others do not count - or at least do not report- less severe complications such as post puncture hematomas or technical complications during the procedure. In addition, there are other differences that might explain the very different figures for the total percentage of complications between the different studies. One of them could be the direct dose/time relationship with the greater risk of hemorrhage that appears in the article by Wang 2020 [21], which explains that doses close to double the pre-established dose were used -10-24 mg for 12-24 hours according to the recommended dosage in the SEATTLE II trial [26]. Other publications attempt to demonstrate the relationship between the dose of fibrinogen and the number of complications. Wayne 2020 [23] performed subgroup analyses based on this dose/n. of complications relationship. Accordingly, the comparison between the conventional strategy according to the SEATTLE II trial (i.e., 24 mg for dual catheters during 4 hours) versus the reduced dose/time strategy (i.e., 8 mg for dual catheters during 4 hours) showed that, although no statistically significant difference was found, in the former group there were 6 bleeding events related to vascular access while in the second group there were no bleeding events. Furthermore, statistically significant results were obtained in terms of reduction of Intensive Care Unit stay and cost with the reduced duration/dosing strategy, without a negative impact on clinical outcomes [23]. In the randomized clinical trial included in the study [18] comparing the use of USCDT vs. Standard CDT, a post hoc sub-analysis of 20 patients who received <8 hours of lysis was performed, and thrombus reduction was higher in the USACDT group ($p = 0.03$).

These results are consistent with the recommendations of the PERT Consortium [3], i.e., smaller dosing strategy for tPA and shorter infusion times for USACDT based on the results of the OPTALYSE PE trial [27]. However, the OPTALYSE PE trial has limitations, including the lack of a control group of patients receiving anticoagulation alone, so the need for future studies is warranted to determine the best approach to the reduced fibrinolytic dose/time strategy with USACDT, which could be an interesting option in the treatment of intermediate-risk PE without the need to increase the risk of complications. It is also worth noting that there are no standardized follow-up protocols, so that post-intervention tests have been performed at different times, and numerous studies emphasize the importance of long-term follow-up. In the article by Klein 2021 [15], after at least 3 months, 73% of patients did not show any signs of RV dysfunction, thus the treatment with USACDT reduced

RV strain not only during the first 24 hours but also in mid-term follow- up in patients with intermediate-high-risk or high-risk PE.

This study has several limitations. Despite the rise of interventional procedures, the data obtained on the efficacy of USACDT in the management of PE in the last two years are scarce and come from studies that do not use a control group. The dose/duration strategy of fibrinolysis with USACDT applied in the different studies is heterogeneous and in some articles the methodology is not very precise, not specifying whether it is performed through a single catheter two. The quantification of complications has been made difficult by the heterogeneity in the qualification and quantification of adverse events. Furthermore, it would be interesting to assess not only the postintervention clinical events but also the medium- and long-term effects in a standardized manner.

Conclusion

Treatment of massive or submassive PE with USACDT reduces RV stress significantly in the short and medium term. The need to combine ultrasound with local thrombolysis, the optimal duration and dose of thrombolysis, and the benefit of USACDT versus anticoagulation alone or in combination with other catheter-directed techniques in intermediate-risk PE would be relevant points to examine in the future. Further controlled prospective studies concerning these issues that are needed.

References

[1] Centers for Disease Control and Prevention (CDC). (2012). Venous thromboembolism in adult hospitalizations - United States, 2007-2009. *MMWR. Morbidity and Mortality Weekly Report*, 61(22), 401–404.

[2] Barnes G. D., Kabrhel, C., Courtney, D. M., Naydenov, S., Wood, T., Rosovsky, R., Rosenfield, K., Giri, J. National PERT Consortium Research Committee. Diversity in the pulmonary embolism response team model: an organizational survey of the National PERT Consortium members. *Chest.* 2016;150:1414–1417.

[3] Rivera-Lebron, B., McDaniel, M., Ahrar, K., Alrifai, A., Dudzinski, D. M., Fanola, C., Blais, D., Janicke, D., Melamed, R., Mohrien, K., Rozycki, E., Ross, C. B., Klein, A. J., Rali, P., Teman, N. R., Yarboro, L., Ichinose, E., Sharma, A. M., Bartos, J. A., ERT Consortium. (2019). Diagnosis, treatment and follow up of acute pulmonary embolism: Consensus practice from the PERT consortium. *Clinical and Applied*

Thrombosis/Hemostasis, 25, 1076029619853037. https://doi.org/10.1177/1076029619853037.

[4] Jaff, M. R., McMurtry, M. S., Archer, S. L., Cushman, M., Goldenberg, N., Goldhaber, S. Z., Jenkins, J. S., Kline, J. A., Michaels, A. D., Thistlethwaite, P., Vedantham, S., White, R. J., Zierler, B. K., American Heart Association Council on Cardiopulmonary, Critical Care, Perioperative and Resuscitation, American Heart Association Council on Peripheral Vascular Disease, & American Heart Association Council on Arteriosclerosis, Thrombosis and Vascular Biology. (2011). Management of massive and submassive pulmonary embolism, iliofemoral deep vein thrombosis, and chronic thromboembolic pulmonary hypertension: a scientific statement from the American Heart Association: A scientific statement from the American heart association. *Circulation,* 123(16), 1788–1830. https://doi.org/10.1161/CIR.0b013e318214914f.

[5] Konstantinides, S. V., Meyer, G., Becattini, C., Bueno, H., Geersing, G. J., Harjola, V. P., Huisman, M. V., Humbert, M., Jennings, C. S., Jiménez, D., Kucher, N., Lang, I. M., Lankeit, M., Lorusso, R., Mazzolai, L., Meneveau, N., Áinle, F. N., Prandoni, P., Pruszczyk, P., The Task Force for the diagnosis and management of acute pulmonary embolism of the European Society of Cardiology (ESC). (2019). 2019 ESC Guidelines for the diagnosis and management of acute pulmonary embolism developed in collaboration with the European Respiratory Society (ERS): The Task Force for the diagnosis and management of acute pulmonary embolism of the European Society of Cardiology (ESC): The Task Force for the diagnosis and management of acute pulmonary embolism of the European Society of Cardiology (ESC). *The European Respiratory Journal: Official Journal of the European Society for Clinical Respiratory Physiology*, 54(3), 1901647. https://doi.org/10.1183/13993003.01647-2019.

[6] Stein, P. D., Matta, F., Janjua, M., Yaekoub, A. Y., Jaweesh, F., & Alrifai, A. (2010). Outcome in stable patients with acute pulmonary embolism who had right ventricular enlargement and/or elevated levels of troponin I. *The American Journal of Cardiology*, 106(4), 558–563. https://doi.org/10.1016/j.amjcard.2010.03.071.

[7] Stein, P. D., & Matta, F. (2012). Thrombolytic therapy in unstable patients with acute pulmonary embolism: saves lives but underused. *The American Journal of Medicine*, 125(5), 465–470. https://doi.org/10.1016/j.amjmed.2011.10.015.

[8] Meyer, G., Vicaut, E., Danays, T., Agnelli, G., Becattini, C., Beyer-Westendorf, J., Bluhmki, E., Bouvaist, H., Brenner, B., Couturaud, F., Dellas, C., Empen, K., Franca, A., Galiè, N., Geibel, A., Goldhaber, S. Z., Jimenez, D., Kozak, M., Kupatt, C., Konstantinides, S. V. (2014). Fibrinolysis for patients with intermediate-risk pulmonary embolism. *The New England Journal of Medicine,* 370(15), 1402–1411. https://doi.org/10.1056/nejmoa1302097.

[9] Goldhaber, S. Z., Haire, W. D., Feldstein, M. L., Miller, M., Toltzis, R., Smith, J. L., Taveira da Silva, A. M., Come, P. C., Lee, R. T., & Parker, J. A. (1993). Alteplase versus heparin in acute pulmonary embolism: randomised trial assessing right-ventricular function and pulmonary perfusion. *Lancet,* 341(8844), 507–511. https://doi.org/10.1016/0140-6736(93)90274-k.

[10] Konstantinides, S., Geibel, A., Heusel, G., Heinrich, F., Kasper, W., & Management Strategies and Prognosis of Pulmonary Embolism-3 Trial Investigators. (2002). Heparin plus alteplase compared with heparin alone in patients with submassive pulmonary embolism. *The New England Journal of Medicine*, 347(15), 1143–1150. https://doi.org/10.1056/NEJMoa021274.

[11] Wu, J., Chen, H., Yu, Y., Peng, L., Li, J., Liang, H., Ba, M., Ruan, H., & Hong, C. (2020). Feasibility of ultrasound-assisted catheter-directed thrombolysis for submassive pulmonary embolism: A meta-analysis of case series. *The Clinical Respiratory Journal*, 14(5), 430–439. https://doi.org/10.1111/crj.13155.

[12] Pei, D. T., Liu, J., Yaqoob, M., Ahmad, W., Bandeali, S. S., Hamzeh, I. R., Virani, S. S., Hira, R. S., Lakkis, N. M., & Alam, M. (2019). Meta-analysis of catheter directed ultrasound-assisted thrombolysis in pulmonary embolism. *The American Journal of Cardiology,* 124(9), 1470–1477. https://doi.org/10.1016/j.amjcard.2019.07.040.

[13] Lou, B. H., Wang, L. H., & Chen, Y. (2017). A meta-analysis of efficacy and safety of catheter-directed interventions in submassive pulmonary embolism. *European Review for Medical and Pharmacological Sciences,* 21(1), 184–198.

[14] Kaymaz, C., Akbal, O. Y., Tanboga, I. H., Hakgor, A., Yilmaz, F., Ozturk, S., Poci, N., Turkday, S., Ozdemir, N., & Konstantinides, S. (2018). Ultrasound-assisted catheter-directed thrombolysis in high-risk and intermediate-high-risk pulmonary embolism: A meta-analysis. *Current vascular pharmacology*, 16(2), 179–189. https://doi.org/10.2174/1570161115666170404122535.

[15] Klein, F., Möbius-Winkler, S., Bäz, L., Pfeifer, R., Fritzenwanger, M., Heymel, S., Franz, M., Aftanski, P., Schulze, P. C., & Kretzschmar, D. (2022). EKOSTM Jena experience: Safety, feasibility, and midterm outcomes of percutaneous ultrasound-assisted catheter-directed thrombolysis in patients with intermediate-high-risk or high-risk pulmonary embolism. *Canadian Respiratory Journal: Journal of the Canadian Thoracic Society*, 2022, 7135958. https://doi.org/10.1155/2022/7135958.

[16] Robles, K. E., Armbruster, A. L., Austin, S. E., & Baker, J. N. (2022). Utilization of EKOS in patients with pulmonary embolism. Innovations (Philadelphia, Pa.), 17(1), 30–36. https://doi.org/10.1177/15569845211057882.

[17] Jiang, C., & Xie, M. (2021). Clinical outcomes of intermediate-risk pulmonary embolism across a Northeastern health system: A multi-center retrospective cohort study. *Cureus*, 13(6), e15888. https://doi.org/10.7759/cureus.15888.

[18] Avgerinos, E. D., Jaber, W., Lacomis, J., Markel, K., McDaniel, M., Rivera-Lebron, B. N., Ross, C. B., Sechrist, J., Toma, C., Chaer, R., & SUNSET sPE Collaborators. (2021). Randomized trial comparing standard versus ultrasound-assisted thrombolysis for Submassive Pulmonary Embolism: The SUNSET sPE trial. *JACC. Cardiovascular Interventions,* 14(12), 1364–1373. https://doi.org/10.1016/j.jcin.2021.04.049.

[19] Stępniewski, J., Kopeć, G., Musiałek, P., Magoń, W., Jonas, K., Waligóra, M., Sobczyk, D., & Podolec, P. (2021). Hemodynamic effects of ultrasound-assisted, catheter-directed, very low-dose, short-time duration thrombolysis in acute intermediate-high risk pulmonary embolism (from the EKOS-PL study). *The*

American Journal of Cardiology, 141, 133–139. https://doi.org/10.1016/j.amjcard.2020.11.004.

[20] Kline, T. M., Rodino, A. M., Dorszynski, A., Murray, B., Cicci, J., & Iyer, P. (2021). Ultrasound-assisted catheter-directed thrombolysis versus systemic anticoagulation alone for submassive pulmonary embolism. *Journal of Thrombosis and Thrombolysis,* 52(1), 130–137. https://doi.org/10.1007/s11239-020-02278-2.

[21] Wang, C. C., Lu, C. R., Hsieh, L. C., Lin, Y. K., Chang, K. C., & Hsu, C. H. (2020). Clinical outcomes of patients with intermediate-to-high-risk pulmonary embolism undergoing ultrasound-assisted catheter-based fibrinolysis therapy in a mid-term follow-up period - A retrospective observational study. *Acta Cardiologica Sinica,* 36(5), 493–502. https://doi.org/10.6515/ACS.202009_36(5).20200330A.

[22] Saylan, B., Çalışkan, T., Canoğlu, K., Ulucan, A. E., & Yılmaz, A. T. (2019). Analysis of pulmonary embolism patients treated with EkoSonicTM endovascular system. *Turk Gogus Kalp Damar Cerrahisi Dergisi*, 28(2), 301–307. https://doi.org/10.5606/tgkdc.dergisi.2020.19133.

[23] Wayne, N. B., Davis, G. A., Macaulay, T. E., Beavers, C. J., Messerli, A. W., Dugan, A., & Smyth, S. S. (2020). Reduced dose thrombolysis with ultrasound-facilitated catheter-directed administration for acute pulmonary embolism reduces length of stay. *Journal of Thrombosis and Thrombolysis*, 49(4), 540–544. https://doi.org/10.1007/s11239-019-02009-2.

[24] Beyer, S. E., Shanafelt, C., Pinto, D. S., Weinstein, J. L., Aronow, H. D., Weinberg, I., Yeh, R. W., Secemsky, E. A., & Carroll, B. J. (2020). Utilization and outcomes of thrombolytic therapy for acute pulmonary embolism: A nationwide cohort study. *Chest,* 157(3), 645–653. https://doi.org/10.1016/j.chest.2019.10.049.

[25] Hooks, B., Sharma, V., Taylor, G., Wadhwani, S., & Ehtesham, M. (2020). Outcome measures for acute submassive pulmonary embolisms at a community-based hospital using ultrasound-facilitated, catheter-directed, low-dose fibrinolysis. *Vascular and Endovascular Surgery,* 54(2), 135–140. https://doi.org/10.1177/1538574419885275.

[26] Piazza, G., Hohlfelder, B., Jaff, M. R., Ouriel, K., Engelhardt, T. C., Sterling, K. M., Jones, N. J., Gurley, J. C., Bhatheja, R., Kennedy, R. J., Goswami, N., Natarajan, K., Rundback, J., Sadiq, I. R., Liu, S. K., Bhalla, N., Raja, M. L., Weinstock, B. S., Cynamon, J., SEATTLE II Investigators. (2015). A prospective, single-arm, multicenter trial of ultrasound-facilitated, catheter-directed, low-dose fibrinolysis for acute massive and submassive pulmonary embolism: The SEATTLE II study. *JACC. Cardiovascular Interventions,* 8(10), 1382–1392. https://doi.org/10.1016/j.jcin.2015.04.020.

[27] Tapson, V. F., Sterling, K., Jones, N., Elder, M., Tripathy, U., Brower, J., Maholic, R. L., Ross, C. B., Natarajan, K., Fong, P., Greenspon, L., Tamaddon, H., Piracha, A. R., Engelhardt, T., Katopodis, J., Marques, V., Sharp, A. S. P., Piazza, G., & Goldhaber, S. Z. (2018). A randomized trial of the optimum duration of acoustic pulse thrombolysis procedure in acute intermediate-risk pulmonary embolism: The OPTALYSE PE trial. *JACC. Cardiovascular Interventions*, 11(14), 1401–1410. https://doi.org/10.1016/j.jcin.2018.04.008.

Chapter 5

Subsegmental Pulmonary Embolism: To Treat or Not Treat?

F. J. Pérez García[1,2], MD
and Antonio Jesús Láinez Ramos-Bossini[1,2,3], MD

[1]Department of Radiology,
Hospital Universitario Virgen de las Nieves,
Granada, Spain
[2] Biosanitary Research Institute,
Granada, Spain
[3]Department of Psychiatry, School of Medicine,
University of Granada, Granada, Spain

Abstract

Pulmonary embolism (PE) represents the third leading cause of cardiovascular-related death in the emergency department. Computed tomography pulmonary angiography is the current imaging technique used to diagnose this condition, allowing to detect its location and extension, which may be variable. In fact, these features are essential to determine its severity, along with clinical presentation. It is completely accepted and validated that patients with central forms of PE (i.e., involving the central, main or lobar pulmonary arteries), should receive urgent treatment, either medical or by invasive procedures, depending on PE severity. In the case of more peripheral PEs (i.e., involving subsegmental pulmonary branches), the decision on whether to treat or not is a matter of great controversy in the scientific literature. The aim of this book chapter is to review the studies published on this subject in recent years to determine whether there is current evidence in favor of administering anticoagulation treatment or not in subsegmental forms of PE. To do so, we performed a systematic review searching the main

In: Understanding and Treating Acute Pulmonary Embolism
Editor: James K. Edwards
ISBN: 979-8-88697-149-1

medical databases (PubMed, Web of Science, Scopus, Cochrane) and we collected information on clinical trials, systematic reviews or meta-analyses on the topic.

Keywords: pulmonary embolism, subsegmental, computed tomography

Introduction

Acute pulmonary embolism (PE) is a very important cause of morbidity and mortality worldwide, being the third cause of mortality among cardiovascular diseases, following myocardial infarction and stroke. Despite exact epidemiological data are not available, the incidence of PE in the general population is estimated to be about 60-95 cases per 100000 inhabitants (Bělohlávek et al., 2013; Cohen et al., 2007). Moreover, between 50000 and 200000 deaths are estimated to occur due to PE every year (Torbicki et al., 2008). Remarkably, up to 95% of deaths take place in patients not previously diagnosed of PE (Jiménez Castro et al., 2007). Thus, the administration of anticoagulant therapy or other therapeutic options is beneficial for patients with this disease (class Ia recommendation in the 2019 European Society of Cardiology on PE diagnosis and management guideline) (Konstantinides et al., 2020). In asymptomatic patients in whom PE is diagnosed incidentally, anticoagulation therapy is similarly recommended by the American College of Chest Physicians guideline (weak recommendation with moderate evidence) (Stevens et al., 2021).

The diagnosis of acute PE continues to be a difficult process since the symptoms and signs that patients exhibit are not specific enough and the differential diagnosis to be considered in this scenario is generally broad. With the development of analytical parameters such as D-dimer, which supports the diagnostic suspicion when elevated in serum, and the publication of clinical scores such as the Wells' criteria, an attempt has been made to provide clinicians with standard tools to establish a preliminary diagnosis based on clinical probability. Nevertheless, recent works point out that their incorrect use guided by the clinician's clinical judgment grants similar performance (Láinez-Ramos-Bossini, Moreno-Suárez, Pérez-García, Gálvez-López, Garrido-Sanz, et al, 2020; Láinez-Ramos-Bossini, Moreno-Suárez, Pérez-García, Gálvez-López, Sanz, et al., 2020).

On the other hand, the diagnosis of PE has evolved greatly in recent years. Since the 1990s, there has been a great technical development of multislice computed tomography (CT), which is currently widely used in the hospital setting. These improvements in radiological equipment have contributed to increase the diagnostic capacity in the study of PE (Rathbun et al., 2000). Previously, helical CT was able to diagnose large central forms of PE but often lacked sufficient definition to detect smaller emboli in more distal arterial branches (Mullins et al., 2000). The technical evolution of multislice CT has progressively allowed to provide sufficient spatial resolution to correctly identify these small filling defects (Láinez Ramos-Bossini AJ, Salmerón Ruiz A, Martínez Barbero JP, Martín Molina JP, Martín Rodríguez JL, López Milena G, Ruiz Santiago F.et al., 2021; Le Gal et al., 2006).

Accordingly, subsegmental PE is defined as isolated or multiple clots that fill the lumen of fifth-order or more distal pulmonary arterial branches. Patients with this type of thrombus may be clinically asymptomatic, paucisymptomatic or, frequently, present pleuritic pain as a consequence of the presence of small peripheral pulmonary infarcts (Donato et al., 2010).

However, this increased diagnostic capacity has not been paralleled by the reduction in mortality that might be expected. This is well demonstrated in the available literature, with several studies showing a significant reduction in mortality despite an increase of up to 81% in the incidence of PE diagnosis in the United States in recent years (Wiener et al., 2011). This apparent overdiagnosis, in addition to other data such as the relative frequency with which subsegmental PEs are incidentally found in asymptomatic patients or those undergoing a CT scan for other reasons, could support hypotheses such as those of some authors who even proposed a model in which the lung would be a sort of filter for small clots that form physiologically in the body circulation and would eventually resolve without causing symptoms or alterations in pulmonary perfusion (Gurney, 1993). In addition, some recent works point out the important number of false positives subsegmental PEs are diagnosed by CT if strict diagnostic criteria are not followed (Castañer et al., 2022).

In general terms, the decision to administer anticoagulant treatment in this type of patient tends to be made on the basis of additional data such as the presence of cancer or previous thrombotic episodes because it is more likely that in these populations, even a PE of slight systemic or pulmonary repercussion could increase the likelihood of further, more extensive thrombotic episodes. To date, the scientific literature has yielded contradictory results on this topic, and no randomized clinical trials or properly structured cohorts with a sufficient level of evidence to confidently support one strategy or another are available. For this reason, in this review we set out to carry out a systematic search of the most recent scientific evidence available to try to elucidate whether the existence of these subsegmental thromboembolisms should be a sufficient reason to decide on the application of anticoagulant therapeutic measures.

Methods

Eligibility Criteria

For the design of this systematic review, we took into account the results obtained in the successive reviews published in the Cochrane Library on this topic in 2012, 2014, 2016, and 2020 (Yoo et al., 2020). The absence of randomized clinical trials described in these works prompted us to broaden our search to include prospective cohort-type studies. We also conducted a search including randomized controlled trials (RCTs), quasi-RCTs (RCTs where allocation to treatment is established by alternation, use of alternate medical records, date of birth or other predictable methods), and controlled clinical trials (CCTs).

The Preferred Reporting Items for Systematic Reviews and Meta-Analyses (PRISMA) guidelines were followed. The design of the systematic review and the selection criteria were based on the PICO search strategy. The population was formed by asymptomatic or symptomatic patients with subsegmental PE (detected by computed tomography pulmonary angiography (CTPA); multi-detector computed tomography; pulmonary digital angiography; or pulmonary arteriograms; the intervention was the use of anticoagulant therapy; the comparator is placebo; and the outcomes included recurrency of a thromboembolic event in a six-month period, minor or major bleeding event and all-cause mortality.

Inclusion Criteria

The inclusion criteria were the following: published RCTs on anticoagulant therapy versus placebo for patients with subsegmental PE which included quantitative results on at least one of the primary outcomes on both arms. The only exclusion criterion was the presence of PE in locations other than subsegmental arteries. Subsegmental PE was defined as “a contrast defect in a subsegmental artery, that is, the first arterial branch division of any segmental artery independent of artery diameter, visible in at least two subsequent axial slices, using a computed tomography scanner with a desired maximum collimator width of $\leq$ 1 mm," as established by the recent definition criteria stated by an international board of thoracic radiologists and VTE specialists (den Exter et al., 2020).

Information Sources and Search Strategy

Two authors searched the PubMed database. Different search strategies were used to optimize the number of relevant outcomes, including keywords such as "pulmonary embolism" and "pulmonary embolism," "subsegmental" or "diagnosis," using several combinations to increase the sensitivity of the search. The following filters were used: abstract and full text available since January 1, 2020. No language restriction was established. The search was updated to March 24, 2022.

Both researchers screened the studies identified in the literature search. Then, they extracted data in an independent fashion and any potential discrepancies were solved by discussion. A standard form was used in order to extract the following data: characteristics of the study (design and method of randomisation); participants; interventions and outcomes (types of outcome measures and adverse events).

Results and Discussion

Our systematic research showed that there are no randomized clinical trials on the management of subsegmental PE available to date. The most relevant systematic review in this regard, conducted by Yoo HHB et al., and published in the Cochrane Library in 2014, which was expanded and updated in 2020 (Yoo et al., 2020), revealed similar results. Of note, there is an ongoing multicenter clinical trial in hospitals in Switzerland, Canada, and the Netherlands that will complete the patient selection phase in February 2024 (Baumgartner et al., 2020). Nevertheless, we included the most relevant recent studies in order to provide evidence in line with the current recommendations on the subject of the review.

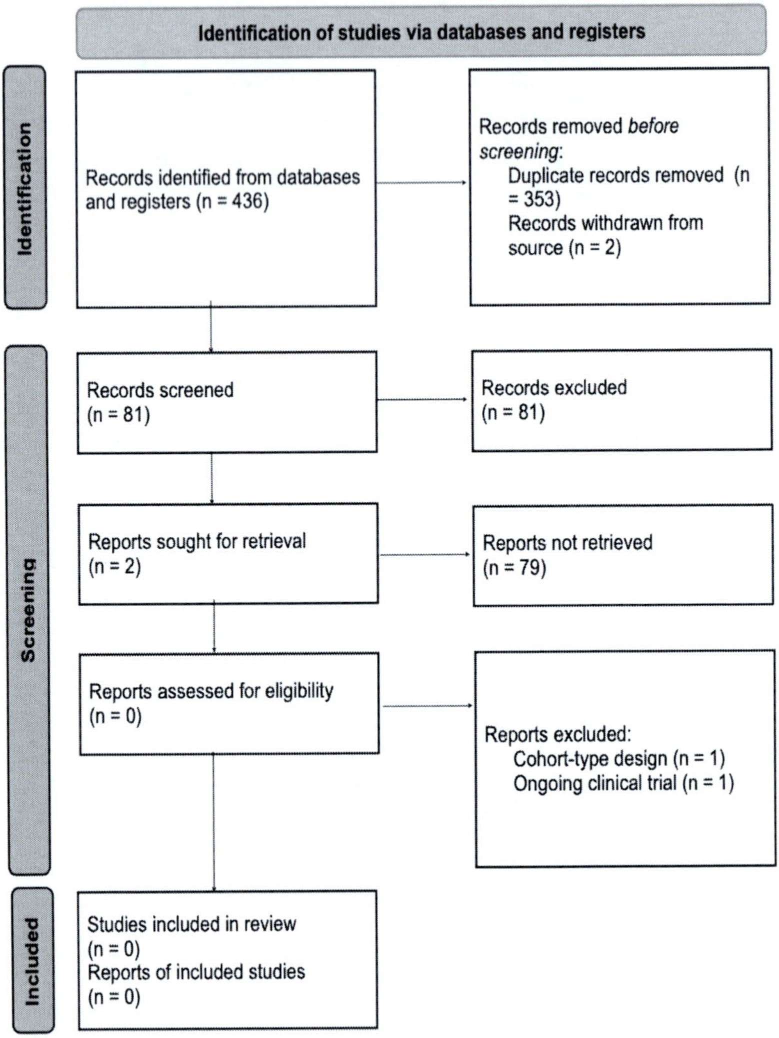

Figure 1. Flow diagram depicting the search conducted in this review.

As mentioned in the introduction, there is a notable lack of knowledge and controversy within the scarce available evidence on the subject, which is logically echoed in the recommendations issued in some of the most important clinical guidelines, such as that of the European Society of Cardiology in collaboration with the European Respiratory Society in 2019, which tends to adopt a conservative view regarding subsegmental PE. This is illustrated by the fact that it is recommended to consider the possibility of a false positive diagnosis in the event that a CT scan shows findings compatible with subsegmental PE, and to assess the need for other imaging tests in such cases (although with weak strength of recommendation, i.e., class IIb C). In addition, it is recommended to accept the diagnosis of PE when a filling defect is found on CT at the segmental level or more proximal in a patient with medium-high clinical probability (class IB recommendation) (Konstantinides et al., 2020).

It should be noted that subsegmental PE is given relevance in the context of patients with concurrent cancer who are incidentally diagnosed with PE. In these patients, it is recommended to initiate treatment in the same way as if the PE was symptomatic, particularly in three scenarios: a PE involving segmental or more proximal arterial branches, a PE involving multiple subsegmental branches, or the existence of an isolated subsegmental PE in association with DVT (class IIa B recommendation). Thus, in the case of patients suffering from cancer, experts advise adopting a therapeutic approach. However, in the case of non-cancer patients, the recommendations of the aforementioned guideline and others (e.g., the American College of Chest Physicians) suggest performing clinical follow-up in selected patients diagnosed with subsegmental PE without associated DVT (class IIC recommendation in the 2021 version) (Stevens et al., 2021). Such recommendation is somewhat consistent with the results observed in works such as the study conducted by Li J et al., (2021), who observed no significant differences in terms of VTE recurrence or adverse events in a prospective study including 48 patients (Li et al., 2021).

Despite these data and the considerable volume of evidence in favor of a more conservative approach in this regard, our experience in the hospital setting is more similar to that presented by Daila T et al., (2020): patients diagnosed with subsegmental PE frequently receive anticoagulation, either because of the association of symptoms or the existence of other risk factors for the recurrence of thrombotic phenomena (Daila et al., 2020). A very recent international prospective cohort study conducted by Le Gal et al., (Le Gal et al., 2022) is of particular value. The authors investigated the recurrence of both deep vein and pulmonary thromboembolic phenomena in an initial sample of 292 patients diagnosed with isolated or multiple subsegmental PE who underwent ultrasound to detect DVT at baseline and 5, 6 or 7 days later. After excluding patients with DVT at the initial or second ultrasound, 266 patients were finally included in the study. Of these, 8 had new episodes of VTE in the 90-day follow-up period: 4 were diagnosed with PE and 4 with DVT, giving a cumulative incidence of 3.1% (95% CI, 1.6% to 6.1%). This is significantly higher than the expected incidence in this type of patient (around 1%), although similar to that observed in patients with PE treated with anticoagulant therapy (Carrier et al., 2010). Therefore, the results of this study (the only prospective one with a large sample to date) support the adoption of a more aggressive strategy in these patients. However, the absence of randomized clinical trials and further prospective studies markedly limits the strength of evidence for recommendations in this regard.

In summary, the current available evidence seems to indicate that there is some clinical benefit of anticoagulation therapy in patients diagnosed with subsegmental PE, in view of the increased likelihood of VTE recurrence observed in recent studies.

Pulmonary Embolism in Patients with COVID-19

An increased relative risk of thromboembolic events in association with SARS-CoV-2 disease (COVID-19) has been widely observed and documented in the literature in recent years (Tan et al., 2021; Ooi et al., 2020). The pathophysiological processes behind this association are only partially understood, although they are thought to include immune-mediated phenomena related to "thromboinflammation" triggered by viral infection, with serum elevation of procoagulant factors (e.g., Von Willebrand factor) to which the "classical" risk factors for venous thrombosis, namely bed rest, hypoxemia or the introduction of catheters, are frequently added.

The incidence of PE in patients with COVID-19 has been estimated in several recent meta-analyses, with values ranging from 12% (Porfidia et al., 2020) to 16.5% (Suh et al., 2021), although there is notable heterogeneity in the results of the studies included, and the multivariate analyses performed in some of these works point to a significant relationship between the incidence of PE and a high degree of disease severity.

In the review by Suh et al., an association with DVT was found in 42.4% of patients. The anatomical location of the PE was frequently not specified in many of the studies, but taking into account the analyses performed, there seems to be a predominantly peripheral location (60.4% of PE in peripheral arteries while 39% were in central arteries). Similar results were obtained in other meta-analyses (18.8% of PTE in main or lobar arteries vs 6.8% of PE in segmental or sub-segmental arteries, $p < 0.001$) (Roncon et al., 2020). In this case, there is little controversy about the need to administer anticoagulant treatment in patients with subsegmental PE, given that, even in patients with

COVID-19 who have not presented a thromboembolic phenomenon, the main clinical guidelines propose the use of anticoagulant drugs (non-fractionated or low molecular weight heparin), frequently in prophylactic doses (Moores et al., 2022).

Therefore, in the case of a COVID-19 patient diagnosed with subsegmental PE, the guidelines generally indicate the administration of anticoagulant therapy, in a similar way to that indicated for patients with active cancer.

Limitations

This review found no randomized clinical trials that provide sufficient evidence to recommend the administration of anticoagulation therapy or only clinical follow-up in patients diagnosed with subsegmental PTE. For this reason, we have had important limitations and have preferred to structure the content in a way that summarizes the most recent state of the art evidence with some of the most relevant studies published to date, although these did not meet the requirements established in the systematic search of the review.

Conclusion

Anticoagulation is not a harmless therapeutic strategy for patients with PE. It carries potential risks and complications that can lead to significant morbidity and mortality. For this reason, as in many other clinical problems, robust evidence supporting patient management is required.

The decision to administer anticoagulant therapy has classically been a source of controversy among clinicians because of the potential controversies related to the clinical benefit-risk balance it poses.

There seems to be greater uniformity of criteria in selected cases such as cancer patients or, as we have seen in recent years, in patients with active SARS-CoV-2 infection. In these cases the administration of anticoagulants is generally recommended.

Outside these selected cases there also seems to be a certain tendency in daily clinical activity to anticoagulate patients with subsegmental PE and the latest published studies point in this direction. According to these studies, despite being peripheral and often having little clinical impact, subsegmental

PE carries a risk of VTE recurrence that is sufficient to recommend anticoagulation for its potential benefit, despite its possible risks.

However, the studies supporting current evidence in this regard are very few, of insufficient sample size, and lack robust designs that would allow these recommendations to be given acceptable confidence. There is at least one international randomized clinical trial in progress and more studies with adequate design and sample are required to provide contrasted information on this clinical problem.

References

Baumgartner, C., Klok, F. A., Carrier, M., Limacher, A., Moor, J., Righini, M., Beer, J.-H., Peluso, M., Rakovic, D., Huisman, M. V., & Aujesky, D. (2020). Clinical Surveillance vs. Anticoagulation For low-risk patiEnts with isolated SubSegmental Pulmonary Embolism: Protocol for a multicentre randomised placebo-controlled non-inferiority trial (SAFE-SSPE). *BMJ Open*, *10*(11), e040151. https://doi.org/10.1136/bmjopen-2020-040151.

Bělohlávek, J., Dytrych, V., & Linhart, A. (2013). Pulmonary embolism, part I: Epidemiology, risk factors and risk stratification, pathophysiology, clinical presentation, diagnosis and nonthrombotic pulmonary embolism. *Experimental & Clinical Cardiology*, *18*(2), 129–138.

Carrier, M., Le Gal, G., Wells, P. S., & Rodger, M. A. (2010). Systematic review: Case-fatality rates of recurrent venous thromboembolism and major bleeding events among patients treated for venous thromboembolism. *Annals of Internal Medicine*, *152*(9), 578–589. https://doi.org/10.7326/0003-4819-152-9-201005040-00008.

Castañer, E., Gonzalez, A., Andreu, M., Lozano, C., & Gallardo, X. (2022). Influence of using recommended radiological criteria on MDCT-angiography diagnosis of single isolated subsegmental pulmonary embolism. *European Radiology*. https://doi.org/10.1007/s00330-021-08480-x.

Cohen, A. T., Agnelli, G., Anderson, F. A., Arcelus, J. I., Bergqvist, D., Brecht, J. G., Greer, I. A., Heit, J. A., Hutchinson, J. L., Kakkar, A. K., Mottier, D., Oger, E., Samama, M.-M., Spannagl, M., & VTE Impact Assessment Group in Europe (VITAE). (2007). Venous thromboembolism (VTE) in Europe. The number of VTE events and associated morbidity and mortality. *Thrombosis and Haemostasis*, *98*(4), 756–764.

Dalia, T., Ranka, S., Patel, N., Lippmann, M., Pierpoline, M., Robinson, A., Hacker, E., Isom, N., Buechler, T., Mabry, T., Janish, C., Satterwhite, L., & Gupta, K. (2020). Clinical presentation and outcomes of patients with isolated subsegmental pulmonary embolism: A tertiary care center experience. *Vascular Medicine (London, England)*, *25*(5), 468–470. https://doi.org/10.1177/1358863X20930279.

den Exter, P. L., Kroft, L. J. M., Gonsalves, C., Le Gal, G., Schaefer-Prokop, C. M., Carrier, M., Huisman, M. V., & Klok, F. A. (2020). Establishing diagnostic criteria and treatment of subsegmental pulmonary embolism: A Delphi analysis of experts.

Research and Practice in Thrombosis and Haemostasis, *4*(8), 1251–1261. https://doi.org/10.1002/rth2.12422.

Donato, A. A., Khoche, S., Santora, J., & Wagner, B. (2010). Clinical outcomes in patients with isolated subsegmental pulmonary emboli diagnosed by multidetector CT pulmonary angiography. *Thrombosis Research*, *126*(4), e266-270. https://doi.org/10.1016/j.thromres.2010.07.001.

Gholamrezanezhad, A., Assadi, M., & Jadvar, H. (2021). *Radiology–Nuclear Medicine Diagnostic Imaging: A Correlative Approach*. Wiley.

Gurney, J. W. (1993). No fooling around: Direct visualization of pulmonary embolism. *Radiology*, *188*(3), 618–619. https://doi.org/10.1148/radiology.188.3.8351321.

Jiménez Castro, D., Sueiro, A., Díaz, G., Escobar, C., García-Rull, S., Picher, J., Taboada, D., & Yusen, R. D. (2007). Prognostic significance of delays in diagnosis of pulmonary embolism. *Thrombosis Research*, *121*(2), 153–158. https://doi.org/10.1016/j.thromres.2007.03.028.

Konstantinides, S. V., Meyer, G., Becattini, C., Bueno, H., Geersing, G.-J., Harjola, V.-P., Huisman, M. V., Humbert, M., Jennings, C. S., Jiménez, D., Kucher, N., Lang, I. M., Lankeit, M., Lorusso, R., Mazzolai, L., Meneveau, N., Ní Áinle, F., Prandoni, P., Pruszczyk, P., … ESC Scientific Document Group. (2020). 2019 ESC Guidelines for the diagnosis and management of acute pulmonary embolism developed in collaboration with the European Respiratory Society (ERS). *European Heart Journal*, *41*(4), 543–603. https://doi.org/10.1093/eurheartj/ehz405.

Láinez-Ramos-Bossini, A. J., Moreno-Suárez, S., Pérez-García, M. C., Gálvez-López, R., Sanz, F. G., & Rivera-Izquierdo, M. (2020). Tromboembolismo pulmonar agudo: Adecuación del manejo de pacientes según las guías de práctica clínica en el servicio de urgencias [*Acute pulmonary thromboembolism: Adequacy of patient management according to clinical practice guidelines in the emergency department*]. *Radiología*. https://doi.org/10.1016/j.rx.2020.06.004.

Láinez-Ramos-Bossini, A. J., Moreno-Suárez, S., Pérez-García, M. del C., Gálvez-López, R., Garrido-Sanz, F., & Rivera-Izquierdo, M. (2020). Use of clinical probability scores and D-dimer in suspected pulmonary embolism. Results from a Spanish retrospective study. *European Journal of Emergency Medicine*, *27*(6), 468–469. https://doi.org/10.1097/MEJ.0000000000000722.

Le Gal, G., Kovacs, M. J., Bertoletti, L., Couturaud, F., Dennie, C., Hirsch, A. M., Huisman, M. V., Klok, F. A., Kraaijpoel, N., Mallick, R., Pecarskie, A., Pena, E., Phillips, P., Pichon, I., Ramsay, T., Righini, M., Rodger, M. A., Roy, P.-M., Sanchez, O., … SSPE Investigators. (2022). Risk for Recurrent Venous Thromboembolism in Patients With Subsegmental Pulmonary Embolism Managed Without Anticoagulation: A Multicenter Prospective Cohort Study. *Annals of Internal Medicine*, *175*(1), 29–35. https://doi.org/10.7326/M21-2981.

Le Gal, G., Righini, M., Parent, F., van Strijen, M., & Couturaud, F. (2006). Diagnosis and management of subsegmental pulmonary embolism. *Journal of Thrombosis and Haemostasis: JTH*, *4*(4), 724–731. https://doi.org/10.1111/j.1538-7836.2006.01819.x.

Li, J., Rolfe-Vyson, V., Rowland, V., Woulfe, T., & Merriman, E. (2021). Management of Single Subsegmental Pulmonary Embolism—A Prospective Observational Study at

North Shore and Waitakere Hospitals, Auckland. *Internal Medicine Journal*. https://doi.org/10.1111/imj.15531.

Moores, L. K., Tritschler, T., Brosnahan, S., Carrier, M., Collen, J. F., Doerschug, K., Holley, A. B., Iaccarino, J., Jimenez, D., LeGal, G., Rali, P., & Wells, P. (2022). Thromboprophylaxis in Patients With COVID-19: A Brief Update to the CHEST Guideline and Expert Panel Report. *CHEST*, *0*(0). https://doi.org/10.1016/j.chest.2022.02.006.

Mullins, M. D., Becker, D. M., Hagspiel, K. D., & Philbrick, J. T. (2000). The role of spiral volumetric computed tomography in the diagnosis of pulmonary embolism. *Archives of Internal Medicine*, *160*(3), 293–298. https://doi.org/10.1001/archinte.160.3.293.

Ooi, M. W. X., Rajai, A., Patel, R., Gerova, N., Godhamgaonkar, V., & Liong, S. Y. (2020). Pulmonary thromboembolic disease in COVID-19 patients on CT pulmonary angiography—Prevalence, pattern of disease and relationship to D-dimer. *European Journal of Radiology*, *132*, 109336. https://doi.org/10.1016/j.ejrad.2020.109336.

Porfidia, A., Valeriani, E., Pola, R., Porreca, E., Rutjes, A. W. S., & Di Nisio, M. (2020). Venous thromboembolism in patients with COVID-19: Systematic review and meta-analysis. *Thrombosis Research*, *196*, 67–74. https://doi.org/10.1016/j.thromres.2020.08.020.

Rathbun, S. W., Raskob, G. E., & Whitsett, T. L. (2000). Sensitivity and specificity of helical computed tomography in the diagnosis of pulmonary embolism: A systematic review. *Annals of Internal Medicine*, *132*(3), 227–232. https://doi.org/10.7326/0003-4819-132-3-200002010-00009.

Roncon, L., Zuin, M., Barco, S., Valerio, L., Zuliani, G., Zonzin, P., & Konstantinides, S. V. (2020). Incidence of acute pulmonary embolism in COVID-19 patients: Systematic review and meta-analysis. *European Journal of Internal Medicine*, *82*, 29–37. https://doi.org/10.1016/j.ejim.2020.09.006.

Stevens, S. M., Woller, S. C., Kreuziger, L. B., Bounameaux, H., Doerschug, K., Geersing, G.-J., Huisman, M. V., Kearon, C., King, C. S., Knighton, A. J., Lake, E., Murin, S., Vintch, J. R. E., Wells, P. S., & Moores, L. K. (2021). Antithrombotic Therapy for VTE Disease: Second Update of the CHEST Guideline and Expert Panel Report. *Chest*, *160*(6), e545–e608. https://doi.org/10.1016/j.chest.2021.07.055.

Suh, Y. J., Hong, H., Ohana, M., Bompard, F., Revel, M.-P., Valle, C., Gervaise, A., Poissy, J., Susen, S., Hékimian, G., Artifoni, M., Periard, D., Contou, D., Delaloye, J., Sanchez, B., Fang, C., Garzillo, G., Robbie, H., & Yoon, S. H. (2021). Pulmonary Embolism and Deep Vein Thrombosis in COVID-19: A Systematic Review and Meta-Analysis. *Radiology*, *298*(2), E70–E80. https://doi.org/10.1148/radiol.2020203557.

Tan, B. K., Mainbourg, S., Friggeri, A., Bertoletti, L., Douplat, M., Dargaud, Y., Grange, C., Lobbes, H., Provencher, S., & Lega, J.-C. (2021). Arterial and venous thromboembolism in COVID-19: A study-level meta-analysis. *Thorax*, *76*(10), 970–979. https://doi.org/10.1136/thoraxjnl-2020-215383.

Torbicki, A., Perrier, A., Konstantinides, S., Agnelli, G., Galiè, N., Pruszczyk, P., Bengel, F., Brady, A. J. B., Ferreira, D., Janssens, U., Klepetko, W., Mayer, E., Remy-Jardin, M., Bassand, J.-P., & ESC Committee for Practice Guidelines (CPG). (2008). Guidelines on the diagnosis and management of acute pulmonary embolism: The Task Force for the Diagnosis and Management of Acute Pulmonary Embolism of the

European Society of Cardiology (ESC). *European Heart Journal*, *29*(18), 2276–2315. https://doi.org/10.1093/eurheartj/ehn310.

Wiener, R. S., Schwartz, L. M., & Woloshin, S. (2011). Time trends in pulmonary embolism in the United States: Evidence of overdiagnosis. *Archives of Internal Medicine*, *171*(9), 831–837. https://doi.org/10.1001/archinternmed.2011.178.

Yoo, H. H., Nunes-Nogueira, V. S., & Fortes Villas Boas, P. J. (2020). Anticoagulant treatment for subsegmental pulmonary embolism. *The Cochrane Database of Systematic Reviews*, *2*, CD010222. https://doi.org/10.1002/14651858.CD010222.pub4.

Index

A

B

C

D

M

O

P

R

S